Love Addiction in Couples Therapy

Toby Morrill

Abstract

Addiction is among the most ubiquitous of mental health issues (Thege et al., 2016; Sussman et al., 2011), priming individuals for relationship distress and comorbid disorders (Bhatia & Davila, 2017; Whisman & Baucom, 2012). The popular medical model of conceptualizing addiction has paved the way for treatment options that are largely short term and focused on symptom management (Fletcher et al., 2015), and couples work is often considered counterproductive in early treatment or delayed until the partner struggling with addiction has had time to prioritize individual treatment. However, high rates of relapse (National Institute on Drug Abuse [NIDA], 2019) and burgeoning cross-addictions (Thege et al., 2016) suggest most current popular treatment approaches are failing to address the root causes of addiction. As rates of addiction continue to increase, it is imperative that therapists more readily access an attachment framework for conceptualizing and treating the biopsychosocial roots of this mental health issue. Intensive short-term dynamic psychotherapy (ISTDP) has emerged among psychoanalytic communities as one such approach based on attachment, but literature on its application in couples therapy is sparse. This study considered the experiences of ISTDP couples therapists who conceptualize and treat addiction as a defense rooted in insecure attachment bonds. Findings demonstrate that, if the goal of treatment is not only symptom cessation, but also to foster a secure attachment in couples therapy, then addictive behaviors may resolve on their own and with lower chances of relapse because the fuel for the addiction has been resolved.

Table of Contents

Chapter 1: Nature of the Study

The nature of the present study was to explore an attachment approach to treat addiction in couples therapy. This chapter will first outline the background of this study, or that increasing rates of substance and behavioral addictions and cross-addictions, suggest we are failing to treat the root causes of addiction. Meanwhile, a growing body of literature has established a link between insecure attachment and addiction that is not well understood, even as scientific communities now recognize similarities in the psychological and neurobiological underpinnings of attachment and addiction systems. This chapter will then outline the purpose of the study and the theoretical framework for understanding these constructs, and a potential framework for understanding addiction as an attachment disorder. Finally, it will offer insight into the foundational principles of ISTDP, an approach based on attachment, to explore its usefulness in conceptualizing and treating addiction within the very arena that might offer the most significant improvement of attachment healing: couples therapy.

Background

Addiction is not a term easily defined. The word *addiction* is rooted in the Latin term *addictionem* which is translated quite literally to "a devoting" (Burkett & Young, 2012; Rosenthal & Faris, 2019). For centuries, romantic love has often been described in literature and the arts as an addiction and it now seems that psychological and neurobiological studies confirm what we always knew to be true: the love and attachment that arises between committed partners, or parents and children, is likely maintained by the psychological and biological mechanisms common to addiction (Burkett & Young, 2012; Fisher et al., 2016; Hostetler & Ryabinin, 2012; Insel, 2003).

But while medical and psychological communities struggle to conceptualize what constitutes an addiction (Rosenthal & Faris, 2019; Sussman & Sussman, 2011), there is emerging consensus that behavioral addictions and substance addictions are similarly maintained (Liese et al., 2020), and it is clear we are living in a society that struggles increasingly with both. Substance abuse is a growing public health crisis with widespread implications (NIDA, 2018; NIAAA, 2019) and approximately half of the adult population will struggle with one or more excessive behavior in a given year (Thege et al., 2016). With ever expanding accessibility to smartphones, social media, food, substances, and pornography, adults and children are living in a world in which bonds to other humans are readily eclipsed, or even replaced, with bonds to substances and behavioral processes. These behaviors frequently co-occur in individuals and can interact to further complicate diagnosis and treatment.

The popular medical model of addiction has paved the way for treatment options which are largely short-term, symptom targeted, and focused on behavioral interventions (Fletcher et al., 2015). Psychodynamic treatments have historically been considered outside the scope of treatment for substance use (Trub & Campbell, 2018) and the literature on using an attachment approach for treating addiction is scarce (Greenman et al., 2019; Johnson, 2019). What is more, couples' work is often considered counterproductive in early treatment and delayed unnecessarily. Relapse rates are high (Fletcher et al., 2015; NIDA, 2019) and cross-addictions appear readily to demonstrate that the predominant treatment approaches are failing to treat the root causes of addiction (Thege et al., 2016).

In recent years, studies have solidified the relationship between insecure attachment styles and addiction. A growing body of research has demonstrated a strong association between insecure attachment and substance misuse or behavioral addictions such as gambling (Anderson et al., 2019; Delvecchio et al., 2016; Fridman, 2019; Keough et al., 2018), problematic Internet and social media use (Liu et al., 2016; Worsley et al., 2018), online sexual activity and sex addictions

(Benfield, 2018; Whoeler et al., 2018; Bolshinsky & Gelkopf, 2019), eating disorders (Hertz et al., 2012), and smartphone addictions (Kim & Koh, 2018; Xie et al., 2019). Although a body of literature has explored the possibilities of applying attachment interventions in the treatment of addiction issues, there is not yet widespread application of these techniques, no less in couples therapy (Fletcher et al., 2015; Katehakis, 2017; Johnson, 2019a).

Intensive short-term dynamic psychotherapy (ISTDP) has emerged over the past several decades as one such approach utilizing attachment principles to address neurosis, character fragility, and behavioral symptoms (Davanloo, 1987, 1990; Abbass et al., 2013). Originally developed in the 1960s, ISTDP has recently been shown effective in the treatment of addiction (Frederickson et al., 2019). The literature is sparse, however, on the use of ISTDP in couples therapy or in the treatment of addiction. Meanwhile, studies establishing a link between insecure attachment and addiction suggests further research is necessary to fill in these gaps in the literature. This study will attempt to do so by exploring the experiences of ISTDP therapists who conceptualize addiction as rooted in attachment and offer clinical treatment within couples therapy.

Purpose Statement

The objective of the present study was to explore ISTDP as an attachment approach to treat addiction in couples therapy. A growing body of literature has established a strong association between insecure attachment and addiction, while researchers recognize similarities between attachment and addiction and the neurobiological systems of both. Yet the literature is sparse in exploring the use of an attachment framework to conceptualize and treat addiction. This study utilized a phenomenological approach to study the experiences of ISTDP therapists who conceptualize and treat addiction as rooted in attachment. It was the objective of this study to explore and discover principles and constructs that might not only fill in large gaps in the literature regarding ISTDP couples therapy but expand the current understanding of addiction as rooted in attachment and its clinical treatment within couples therapy.

Research Questions

Within both qualitative and quantitative analyses, the premise of each approach is that there is a line of inquiry to be addressed, as was the aim of this study. However, the creation of research questions in a qualitative analysis is inherently different than that in a quantitative analysis. Because, although the processes are similar, a qualitative approach relies on text or image data and involve steps in data analysis unique to a qualitative approach (Creswell & Creswell, 2018).

For this study, the central research question and corresponding subquestions were as follows:

RQ1: What are the perspectives of ISTDP therapists who utilize an attachment approach to treat addiction in couples therapy?

SRQ1: How do ISTDP therapists conceptualize the etiology and maintenance of addiction?

SRQ2: How do ISTDP therapists conceptualize treatment goals for couples in addiction?

SRQ3: How do the experiences of ISTDP couples therapists inform the use of an attachment approach to treat addiction in couples therapy?

Theoretical Framework

The Neurobiology of Attachment and Addiction

In recent years, researchers have begun to recognize similarities between attachment systems and addictions not only on a psychological level, but on a neurobiological level as well. Neuroscientists and clinical psychologists have now integrated research in order to map out the neural circuitry that underlies emotional bonds, while advancements in neuroscience now show that attachment will impact the development, structure, and functioning of the brain (Cihan et al., 2014). In infancy, a child has few neural connections outside the most basic two neural structures that, along with the automatic nervous system, signal basic needs such as hunger, thirst, and fear (Cihan et al., 2014). When an attentive caregiver responds to an infant's cues by satisfying needs, the child's automatic nervous system is regulated simultaneously with the central nervous system. As the infant's emotions are regulated by a caregiver, the infant's brain then develops new neural pathways which are strengthened each and every time the caregiver meets the infant's needs in a timely manner. Combined with mirroring, the caregiver's actions thereby provide "the scaffolding upon which the infant's right brain is built" (Cihan et al., 2014, p. 533). Eventually the neurochemical changes of a close attachment relationship offer an experience evolutionary wired to be pleasurable for both parties involved. Interactions between a caregiver and infant then continue to strengthen neural pathways and the neurotransmitter "high" that occurs is eventually sought for nothing more than the pleasure of its experience. Humans are thus neurobiologically wired to need secure attachment bonds offering safety and emotional availability during stress throughout our lifetime.

Neurologists have also suggested that attachment and addiction share common neurobiological structures, as there is evidence that addictive substances and social engagement with partners activate and alter the very same neurotransmitter mechanisms (Burkett & Young, 2012; Hostetler & Ryabinin, 2012). Feelings of intense love have been shown to engage the same dopamine-rich "reward center" regions of the brain that are also activated in addiction to substances and behavioral processes. Social attachment, it turns out, will engage the brain's dopamine rich reward system that plays an integral role in maintaining addictive behaviors (Acevedo & Aron, 2009; Fisher et al., 2016). In fact, the chemical released in the brain during close attachment resembles that of opiates (Insel, 2003) and even thinking about a loved on appears

to stimulate brain activity patterns similar to those that activate after the ingestion of cocaine or

other opiates (Bartles & Zeki, 2000). Rejection cues, on the other hand, are processed in the same

area of the brain as physical pain, demonstrating that disconnection is experienced similarly to

physical pain and will generate cues an individual is at risk for having basic needs met

(Eisenberger, 2013). Even at a neurological level, then, we see it is the security of one's earliest

attachment relationships that is responsible for a sense of emotional safety and affect regulation.

The Psychology of Attachment and Addiction

Addiction researchers have also repeatedly observed the psychological effects of close

relationship bonds and observed analogous responses to drugs of choice. Studies have identified

strikingly similar patterns of affective, cognitive, and behavioral responses to attachment figures

as to addictive substances (Burkett & Young, 2012). Individuals experience despair or

preoccupation in the absence of attachment figures or loved ones, but feel joy or even euphoria

when reunited with them. Individuals also experience despair or preoccupation in the absence of

addictive substances, but feel joy or even euphoria when they obtain or ingest the drug. These

studies suggest that the psychological and neurobiological mechanisms and processes supporting

addiction are those involved in the maintenance of close relationships (Burkett & Young, 2012;

Insel, 2003) and that insecure relationships might just be a far too often unrecognized factor of

susceptibility to addiction.

Attachment Theory

Attachment theory is one of the most profoundly influential perspectives on human

development. Originally established by John Bowlby in 1969, and later expanded upon by Mary

Ainsworth et al. (1978), attachment theory offers a framework for how early interpersonal relationships shape human psychological functioning throughout the lifespan. Today, decades of research have confirmed that few factors have such profound effect on the individual human regulation of emotion as do close and intimate relationships (Bowlby, 1988).

Attachment theory is primarily based on how the individual self develops in relation to others, with a fundamental focus on how humans seek protection from loved ones when facing stress or danger. Bowlby (1969) developed this theory after observing children separated from their primary caregivers during World War II. In his work, Bowlby noticed that "the young child's hunger for his mother's love and presence is as great as his hunger for food" and that a mother's absence would inevitably elicit from a child "a powerful sense of loss and anger" (Bowlby, 1969, p. xiii). He also observed the child's emotional attachment to his primary caregiver as biologically important because, from an evolutionary standpoint, it is the infant who remains close to its caregiver that is likely to be cared for, remain safe from predators, and survive to eventually reproduce. Ainsworth, originally a colleague of Bowlby's, built upon his research when she observed the behavior of children were separated from, and later reunited with, caregivers (Ainsworth et al., 1978). This research model, entitled the Strange Situation, eventually led to Ainsworth's classification of children as secure or insecure, subcategories of which were later expanded upon with further research.

According to Bowlby (1969, 1988), humans are biologically wired for close and loving bonds with those who ensure support, safety, and connection. The early relationship between child and primary caregiver is thus at the very center of attachment theory. The bond that forms in this relationship becomes the core of a child's identity development, intrapersonal regulation, and interpersonal attitudes, which combined constitute "internal working models" (Bowlby, 1977) of self and others. These are the blueprints this individual will bring into future relationships and the foundation for attachment styles most often today categorized as secure, avoidant, or anxious.

Attachment Styles

According to Bowlby (1969, 1980), it is the experience of attachment security in childhood that is the scaffolding upon which one's mental health and overall well-being is built. Individuals demonstrating *secure* attachment styles are capable of deep and meaningful relationships and can tolerate their own emotions without feeling overwhelmed. They are able to identify their own emotional experience as separate from others and are not overly self-critical. Individuals demonstrating *dismissing* or *avoidant* attachment styles are overly self-reliant and dismiss the value of important attachment relationships because they have learned that relationships are often disappointing or dangerous (Mikulincer et al., 2009). They will minimize their own emotional experience and tend to overidealize or be derogatory towards attachment figures. Finally, *preoccupied* or *anxious* individuals tend to be consumed with relationship loss or abandonment and preoccupied with attachment relationships. They try to minimize anxiety by soliciting love from others but might become upset if they perceive rejection. These individuals also tend to frequently revisit painful attachment memories and their emotional system is often hyperactivated as sadness or anger result (George et al., 1985). Notably, while research has verified attachment-related differences in emotion regulation, these studies repeatedly highlight a need for more research exploring the kinds of therapeutic interventions that might counteract insecure attachment strategies and the effects thereof (Mikulincer & Shaver, 2019).

Attachment in Childhood

Bowlby theorized that an infant who is able to turn to a primary caregiver for physical needs such as food and safety, as well as psychological needs such as love and comfort, will experience secure attachment. This infant will turn to their caregiver as a *safe haven* when experiencing fear or distress and will otherwise explore their surroundings without fear, knowing the caregiver is a *secure base* to which they may return if necessary. The infant whose needs for physical or psychological safety are not met by a primary caregiver, however, will develop a different set of behaviors as a result of not experiencing their caregiver as a safe haven or a secure base. Bowlby theorized that this adaptive set of strategies, while successfully managing immediate distress, would increase vulnerabilities to psychopathology (Bowlby, 1977; Levy & Johnson, 2019). Over many years, an ever growing body of research has validated Bowlby's hypothesis connecting insecure attachment styles to a broad range of child and adult clinical disorders from depression to eating disorders and substance misuse (Delvecchio et al., 2016; Fridman, 2019; Hertz et al., 2012; Madigan et al., 2016; Tasca & Balfour, 2014).

Today, over half a century later, decades of research have led researchers and clinicians to consider the profoundly fundamental role attachment plays in all important relationships from infancy to adulthood (Ainsworth et al., 1978; 1985; Bowlby, 1988). A basic tenant of attachment theory is that an individual will require secure attachment throughout the lifespan, not just in childhood. According to Bowlby, "[a]ll of us, from the cradle to the grave are happiest when life is organized as a series of excursions, long or short, from the secure base provided by our attachment figures" (1988, p. 62). For young children, attachment guarantees survival, while in later human development, the focus of attachment shifts from the physical to the psychological (Holmes, 2015). Therefore, while attachment theory is traditionally based on the relationship between infant and caregiver, modern attachment research is often focused on the secure bonds that exist later in life.

Attachment in Adulthood

Haven and Shaver's (1987) seminal work on adult love as an attachment process analogous to that between child and caregiver has sparked hundreds of empirical studies demonstrating that adults develop strong emotional bonds to their intimate partners that have a profound effect on psychological well-being. As adults, many individuals report that a romantic partner or a parent often serve as a primary attachment figure in life. However, the quality of these attachment relationships can vary significantly from one relationship to the next.

These bonds, when offering security, encourage both independence and emotional closeness. Critically, one who is *securely attached* will use that partner as a *safe haven* in times of distress and also consider them a *safe base* from which to go out and take risks in the world. Just as a securely attached child will take more risks in moving away from the caregiver to explore the environment, so to will a securely attached adult will take more risks exploring their emotional experience in the counseling room and in life beyond. The foundation of secure romantic attachment is accessibility and mutual responsiveness, which can increase both partners' ability to tolerate the stress associated with life circumstances. Secure attachment is linked with positive relationship functioning including trust, commitment, and higher dyadic satisfaction (Kobak & Hazan, 1991). Securely attached partners also exhibit flexible functioning in relationship (Bowlby, 1969, 1982; Delvecchio et al., 2016) and are able to demonstrate more curiosity about their partner and remain open to new information. These relationships encourage optimal experiences that enhance the life of the self and the other.

On the other hand, perceived threats to the attachment bond between partners creates psychological distress. One who is insecurely attached will question whether their partner will be available when needed and will thus be hesitant to depend on them. The insecurely attached adult will not rely on internal representations of attachment figures but instead employ behavioral strategies to override fears and anxieties (Bowlby, 1969, 1982; Delvecchio et al., 2016; Greenman et al., 2019).

Addiction as an Attachment Disorder

Edward Khantzian (1997) was one of the first theorists to suggest that substance misuse should be conceptualized not as a pleasure-seeking behavior, but instead as one to seek comfort and contact when unable to tolerate one's own emotional experience. Höfler and Kooyman (1996) had also theorized why it is that a suffering individual might attach to a substance as an alternative to a relationship. Building upon this theory, it was Flores (2004, 2006) to first suggest addiction should be conceptualized as an attachment disorder outright. According to Flores, it is the individual who finds difficulty in establishing safe intimate relationships who will seek alternative methods to self-soothe when distressed (2004, 2006). As substance use offers a consistent feeling of having a secure base, the use of substances will become an attachment, which thereby protects an individual from relationship vulnerability all while further impeding one's ability to create safe interpersonal relationships (Flores, 2004, 2006).

It is not difficult to view addiction within an attachment framework. In short, attachment allows one to see how an individual who is not taught to regulate affect through human connection will turn to addictive substances or behavioral processes that allow them to do so. Through this lens, it is easy to see why those without secure attachment are more likely to regulate emotions using the immediate and consistent gratification offered by addictive substances (e.g., alcohol or drug use) or addictive behaviors (e.g., porn, smartphone use, or eating disorders) (Benfield, 2018; Molnar et al., 2010). A cyclical relationship then ensues as one experiences relationship distress that leads to addictive coping behaviors and eventually it is the addiction, rather than a partner, that becomes a safe and secure base for the addicted partner. As Flores (2006) succinctly stated, attachment theory looks at addiction as "a consequence and a failed solution to an impaired ability to form healthy emotionally regulating relationships" (p. 6).

While a growing body of literature has solidified the relationship between insecure attachment and addiction (Anderson et al., 2019; Benfield, 2018; Bolshinsky & Gelkopf, 2019; Delvecchio et al., 2016; Hertz et al., 2012; Fridman, 2019; Kim & Koh, 2018; Keough et al., 2018; Liu et al., 2016; Whoeler et al., 2018; Worsley et al., 2018; Xie et al., 2019), few studies have explored the use of attachment informed interventions in the treatment of addiction (Fletcher et al., 2015; Benfield, 2018; Katehakis, 2017). ISTDP exists within psychoanalytic communities as one such approach that, rooted in attachment, might inform the greater psychological community about the critical role of attachment in the clinical treatment of addiction.

Intensive Short-Term Dynamic Psychotherapy (ISTDP)

Initially developed in the 1960s by Habib Davanloo (1987), ISTDP is a form of psychodynamic treatment and set of therapeutic principles based largely on Freud's second theory of anxiety, which could actually be understood as the first attachment theory (Abbass et al., 2013). Davanloo (1990) reported results in a series of longitudinal cases and eventually established guidelines and a theoretical approach for implementing this model. Supported by a growing number of empirical studies, alongside the publication of one meta-analysis (Abbass et al., 2012), ISTDP has been proven to be a highly complex but effective approach to alleviating physical and psychological distress in clinical treatment.

Davanloo (1990) described Freud's belief that the superego becomes established relatively late in developmental history, but he posited that the superego exists much earlier in infancy. Neurotic disturbances thus arise as experiences of trauma disrupt or damage the affectionate bond between child and caretaker, and a child responds to this disruption with sadistic or murderous rage. As a result of feeling murderous rage towards a beloved caretaker, the child naturally experiences guilt and grief which, along with the rage, must be repressed into the unconscious. Symptomatic pathologies then develop as the child grows and attempts to keep feelings repressed and function in manner acceptable to the world in which they must survive. According to foundational tenants of ISTDP, the earlier and more intense the experience of attachment trauma, the more the ego will be trapped between the sadistic id and sadistic superego, and all the more paralyzed the ego will become in managing the resistance of repression demanded by the superego.

Attachment Trauma

According to Davonloo (1990), "The vast majority of neurosis stems from the patient's conflicting feelings within family relationships" (p. 190). While Davanloo explicitly mentioned the importance of attachment bonds affecting psychological development, he refrained from elaborating on the details of this attachment relationship or how attachment ruptures might be characterized. Thus, it is the work of other pioneers in the field of attachment theory discussed above such as Bowlby (1969, 1980, 1988) and Ainsworth (1978) that expanded upon constructs of attachment theory and its application in conceptualizing healthy or unhealthy intrapersonal development and the mental health implications of both.

Theorists suggest many experiences that constitute attachment trauma. While physical, verbal, or sexual abuse in childhood will naturally meet the threshold, studies also show that emotional neglect from a caregiver is equally detrimental to a child's experiences of secure attachment. For instance, French psychoanalyst Andre Green was the first to introduce the term "dead mother" as referring to an unavailable or emotionally absent caregiver. This mother, unable to attune to a child's emotional needs, will elicit from the child repeated, desperate attempts connect with the mother. A child will do anything to connect with a parent, even if that means deadening their own emotional experience in order to join her. This child's experience is a compromising of their own emotional experience that results in emotional dysregulation and the very insecure attachment that renders necessary a reliance on maladaptive behaviors to self-regulate. Notably, ISTDP suggests that untreated attachment trauma will worsen over time as the feelings and behaviors linked to past attachment experiences are reinforced by new traumatic attachment experiences, and it becomes more difficult to link current behaviors to the original attachment traumas (Abbass et al., 2012). Unhealthy coping mechanisms thus become more acute as the dissociation, acting out, or repetitive behaviors become more severe.

The Triangle of Conflict and The Triangle of Persons

Originally conceptualized by Menninger (1958) and expanded upon by Malan (1979), the triangle of conflict (Figure 1) and the triangle of persons (Figure 2) offer a model of intrapsychic conflict foundational to ISTDP. Davanloo (1980, 1990) utilized these triangles to both diagnose and guide interventions in ISTDP. In the three corners of the triangle of conflict (Figure 1) exist *feelings and impulses, anxiety,* and *defense mechanisms.* When core feelings arise that cannot be tolerated, an individual experiences a rise of anxiety along with feeling and employs a defense to discharge feeling and anxiety. Linked to this is the triangle of persons (Figure 2), representing the most significant people in a patient's life towards whom a patient might experience these feelings. In linking these triangles to conceptualize the model of intrapsychic conflict, Coughlin (1996/2018) writes:

Feelings do not exist in a vacuum, but arise both toward and in reaction to others. There is always an interpersonal context to the arousal of emotion, even if only in fantasy. It is hypothesized that those affective states which caretakers did not tolerate will be suffused with anxiety and lead to the operation of a defense. We cannot assume that only certain feelings, such as anger, will be prohibited; for in some families nothing is experienced as more threatening and, therefore, is more heavily prohibited than the expression of tender feelings (pp. 6-7).

Figure 1

Triangle of Conflict

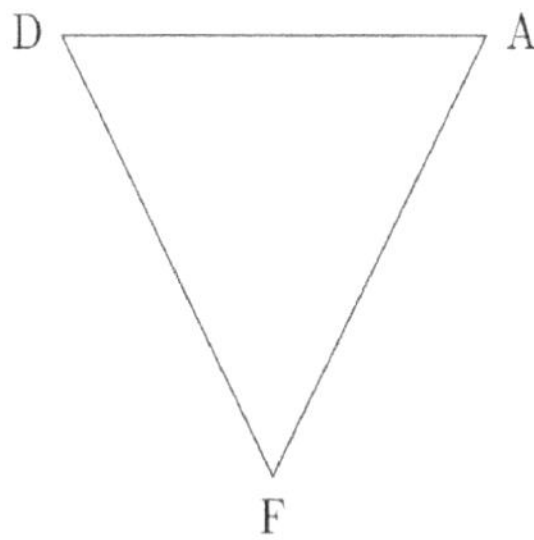

Figure 2

Triangle of Persons

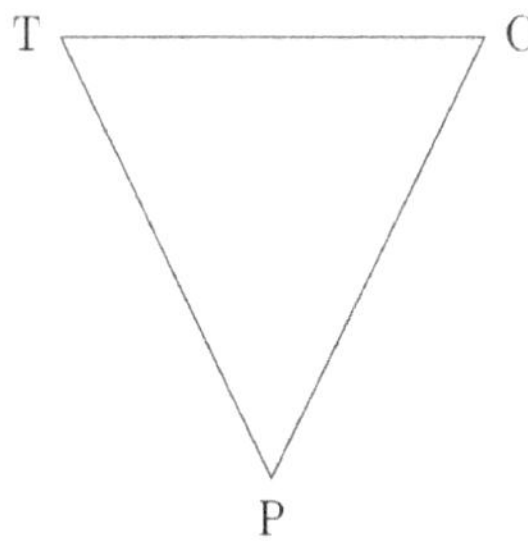

Feelings and Impulses

Core feelings and impulses that one experiences are at the bottom of the triangle which include anger, sadness, fear, joy, disgust, excitement, and sexual desire. Physiological sensations accompany each of these core feelings, whether or not the patient is aware of such somatic experiences. These feelings, as noted above, arise not in a vacuum, but towards other people of significance in a patient's life (Coughlin, 1996/2018).

Anxiety

A critical component of effective treatment in ISTDP is the therapist's ability to help patients regulate their experience of anxiety, which increases notably throughout sessions when the patient's defenses are confronted or blocked. Anxiety may manifest in the patient's body occur in one of four different pathways. First, and healthiest, anxiety might manifest in the striated muscles. This presents in a patient as deep sighing, tensing and clenching of fists, or even fidgeting. Second, anxiety might manifest in the sympathetic nervous system. This presents in a patient as a racing heart, sweating, or dry mouth. Third, anxiety might manifest in the parasympathetic nervous system, or the smooth muscle. This presents in a patient as gastrointestinal symptoms such as nausea, dizziness, diarrhea, acid reflux, or loss of muscle tension. Fourth, and finally, anxiety might manifest in cognitive perceptual disruption. This presents in a patient as incoherent or racing thoughts, tunnel vision, or other visual or auditory disturbances.

Critically, a patient experiencing symptoms in the last two categories, smooth muscle or cognitive perceptual functioning, will have exceeded their window of tolerance and can no longer regulate anxiety in a healthy manner. This patient will experience somatic or depressive symptoms that render the establishment of a therapeutic alliance difficult. On the other hand, a patient experiencing anxiety at the lowest levels will employ destructive defenses that prevent healthy emotional experiences in intimate relationships. It is thus the job of the ISTDP therapist to recognize when a patient has gone over the threshold of experiencing anxiety safely in the body and should intervene to reduce anxiety (Frederickson, 2013; Have-de Labije & Neborsky, 2012). ISTDP clinicians are trained to carefully monitor a patient's somatic experiences of anxiety (Frederickson, 2013) in order to work within the optimal "window of tolerance" (Siegel, 1999).

Most therapies will aim to reduce anxiety. ISTDP will differ as the therapist becomes a biofeedback loop for the patient and encourages recognizing anxiety as a sign of feelings on the rise. As an ISTDP therapist challenges the use of defense mechanisms in session, the therapist must monitor which feelings trigger anxiety in real time and bring these to the attention of the patient. A neuroscientific perspective offered by Neborsky & Lewis (2011) offers insight into changes that happen during this biofeedback loop. Attentiveness will stimulate synaptic growth such that a patient learns to engage the cortex to separate anxiety from emotions. This leads to a more 'attentive ego' promoting cortical inhibition of the amygdala so that patients can pay attention to the somatic and cognitive experiences of anxiety and become curious about the emotions that underlie the anxiety. Neural circuitry once damaged by traumatic experiences are actually able to be restored.

Defense Mechanisms

Early on, children will learn to identify what emotions threaten their acceptability to a caregiver. For example, if a child approaches a parent for comfort when the child is angry or sad, and the parent rejects the child in their distressed sate, a child will learn to hide such emotions even from the self. Over time anxiety replaces these emotions. ISTDP is founded on the principle that these early ruptures in the bond between child and caregiver lead to a myriad of complex and often undesirable feelings that are suppressed from awareness by *anxiety* and *defense mechanisms*.

These defense mechanisms, once necessary for survival as children, become incorporated into all interpersonal relationships developed throughout the lifespan. In other words, individuals in adult relationships continue to employ the same defense mechanisms once used to survive childhood because they are part of that individual's blueprint for relationship functioning. However, because these defense mechanisms are actually maladaptive to healthy emotional regulation, they begin to cause problems as it is then the conflict between unconscious feelings and impulses, and the defenses constructed to protect them, leads to symptoms including undesirable behaviors, psychiatric disorders, and relationship distress (Abbass et al., 2012; Abbass, 2015; Davanloo, 1989).

Therapists trained in ISTDP will work together with a patient to recognize and block these maladaptive defense mechanisms. The framework of ISTDP suggests that *anxiety* in a patient is a signal that some threatening feeling or impulse is on the rise (Abbass et al., 2013). Then the defenses a patient employs will keep threatening feelings out of consciousness. However, it is also the excessive reliance on these defenses causes the very *symptoms* and *difficulties* the patient comes to therapy to address (Abbass et al., 2013). Early in treatment, therefore, a clinician will ideally address the defense mechanisms that keep a patient emotionally distant and encourage a therapeutic intimacy that serves to strengthen the therapeutic alliance and the patient's capacity to tolerate emotional closeness (Frederickson, 2013; Kuhn, 2014). The goal in ISTDP is then to overcome defenses and allow the patient to experience their true emotions (Abbass et al., 2013).

Unconscious Therapeutic Alliance

The collaborative efforts of the ISTDP therapist and patient in blocking these defenses will quickly build the patient's tolerance for feeling and the building of an unconscious therapeutic alliance (UTA), which serves as a powerful force to battle against resistance. As the UTA strengthens to overpower resistance, this will result in what Davanloo (1995) termed the "unlocking of the unconscious" in which underlying emotions are accessible and working through them becomes possible (Abbass et al., 2013; Johansson et al., 2014). In Davanloo's work he demonstrated that more resistant and complex patients require more of the unlocking experiences, but that the adjustment of defenses will often bring about long-lasting changes in the ability to emotionally process experiences (Davanloo, 1980). This entire process of working with a patient using the ISTDP principles is termed the *central dynamic sequence* (Davanloo, 1990).

Theoretical and Operational Definitions

Addiction. A state of psychological or physical dependence (or both) on the use of alcohol, other drugs, or behavioral processes (APA, 2021).

Anxiety. A physiological response; "in ISTDP, anxiety refers to an activation of the biological fear system in response to internal stimuli, which is an extension of what Freud called 'signal anxiety'" (Kuhn, 2014).

Anxiety regulation. A method used to lower a patients' anxiety (Kuhn, 2014)

Attachment. Defined by Bowlby (1969) as a "lasting psychological connectedness between human beings" (p. 194); "the tendency to form such bonds with certain other individuals in infancy as well as the tendency in adulthood to seek emotionally supportive social relationships" (APA, 2021).

Attachment trauma. "Early-life events such as covert or overt abuse, neglect, or loss, which cause damage to the bonds to early attachment figures (e.g., parents, siblings, grandparents)" (Kuhn, 2014, p. 16).

Capacity. See "*ego adaptive capacity.*"

Capacity building. The process of building up capacity within a patient.

Couple. Two partners in a committed relationship.

Complex feelings. A mixture of conflicting positive feelings (e.g., love or appreciation) and negative feelings (e.g., anger) that are generally held towards early and current attachment figures (Kuhn, 2014).

Couple in addiction. Two partners in a committed relationship in which one or both partner struggles with issues of *addiction* as defined herein.

Couples therapy. Therapy in which "both partners in a committed relationship are treated at the same time by the same therapist or therapists" (APA, 2021) and the focus of treatment is on problems within and between the individuals that affect the relationship.

Defense. "Any mechanism used for the avoidance of true feeling" (Davanloo, 2000, p. 113).

Defense restructuring: "replacing regressive or primitive defenses with self-observation and more mature defenses" (Kuhn, 2014, p. 251-252).

Ego adaptive capacity (or *capacity*): a patient's ability to bear anxiety, observe and understand the basics of their inner life (feelings, anxiety, defenses, desires, preferences, etc.) with compassion rather than judgement, and to hold complex feelings and contradictory impulses with acceptance (Kuhn, 2014).

Emotional intimacy (or emotional closeness). "Being direct, honest, authentic, caring, tender, and vulnerable" (Kuhn, 2014, p. 40); a key aspect off attachment, as in the wake of attachment trauma it will provoke *anxiety* (Kuhn, 2014).

Feeling (or *affect*). Primary motivators of human behavior; in ISTDP, *core feelings* are associated with attachment trauma and central to the genesis of psychopathology (Kuhn, 2014).

Impulse. "A specific action tendency associated with a feeling" (Kuhn, 2014, p. 138).

ISTDP. An evidence-based psychotherapy strongly supported by current clinical research studies with interventions specifically designed to "resolve anxiety, depression, somatization and personality disorders, as well as alleviate a variety of self-defeating behaviors, many of which derive from unstable or troubled early life attachments" (California Society for Intensive Short-term Dynamic Psychotherapy, 2021).

ISTDP therapist. A licensed therapist utilizing interventions of *ISTDP* as defined herein.

ISTDP couples therapist. A licensed therapist who works with couples utilizing interventions of *ISTDP* as defined herein.

Restructuring. "A set of techniques intended to bring structural change" (Kuhn, 2014, p. 251) or *build capacity* within a patient.

Threshold. The limit of a patient's ability to use striated muscle discharge pathways for the anxiety that exists within the body (Kuhn, 2014).

Transference. "A patient's tendency to bring aspects of their problematic relationships with early attachment figures into the therapy in ways that simultaneously impede therapy (resistance) and provide therapeutic opportunities" (Kuhn, 2014, p. 316).

Triangle of conflict. A visual to the organize the components of intrapsychic conflict, the three corners of which include underlying (often unconscious) feeling, the anxiety that ensues as a result of the feeling, and the defenses employed to avoid that feeling (Kuhn, 2014).

Summary

Attachment theory is a profoundly influential perspective on human development offering a framework for how early interpersonal relationships shape human psychological functioning throughout the lifespan. Today, decades of research have confirmed that few factors have such a profound effect on the individual human regulation of emotion as do close and intimate relationships. In recent years, research has also established similarities between attachment systems and addictions on a psychological and neurobiological level. Although a growing body of literature has solidified the relationship between insecure attachment and addiction, few studies have explored the use of attachment informed interventions in the treatment addiction, no less within couples therapy.

The following chapter will offer an overview of the term addiction and its development has affected treatment options today. It will then summarize a growing body of research establishing an association between insecure attachment and addiction that still fails to understand the causal direction of this relationship and the treatment implications thereof. Finally, it will examine the gaps in literature regarding the use of ISTDP in couples therapy and consider how the experiences of ISTDP couples therapist might inform greater psychological community about the usefulness of conceptualizing addiction as rooted in attachment and one best addressed in attachment-focused couples therapy.

Chapter 2: Literature Review

This literature review will offer an overview of the term addiction and how the popular disease model has informed treatment options as they exist today. It will then explore a growing body of research that, while establishing an association between insecure attachment and addiction, fails to understand the causal direction of this relationship and the treatment implications thereof. Finally, this review will explore the scarcity of research regarding the use of ISTDP couples therapy, an approach based in attachment, and consider how filling these gaps might inform the treatment of the biopsychosocial roots of addiction in couples therapy.

The Definition of Addiction

A phenomenon that is multidimensional and complex, there is no one-size-fits-all definition of addiction. The American National Institute on Drug Abuse (2018) and the American Psychiatric Association (2019) cite addiction as a brain disease caused by changes in the structure and functioning of the brain, while other researchers argue not enough is known about addiction to label it a disease and question whether it is a mental health issue or even a matter of choice (Heyman, 2013). Although disagreements persist as to whether behaviors casually labeled addictions are better understood as disorders, compulsions, or even manifestations of an underlying disorder (Dalal & Basu, 2016), characteristics common to the term appear easier to agree upon and include substances or behaviors causing altered feelings, preoccupation, temporary satiation, loss of control, and negative consequences (Sussman & Sussman, 2011). The APA (2021) defines addiction as a state of psychological or physical dependence (or both) on the use of alcohol, other drugs, or behavioral processes. Approximately half of adults will struggle with such excessive behaviors and more research is necessary to understand the etiology and effective treatment of these behaviors (Thege et al., 2016).

The *Diagnostic and Statistical Manual of Mental Disorders*, Fifth Edition (*DSM-5*) has evolved in its use of the term addiction (American Psychiatric Association [APA], 2013). While originally precluded from earlier editions as stigmatizing and too difficult to define, the DSM-5 introduced a category of 'Substance-Related and Addictive Disorders' (APA, 2013, p. 483), characterizing substance abuse disorders as a "pathological pattern of behaviors related to the use of the substance" (APA, 2013, p. 483). The text notes, however, that the term addiction is "omitted from the official DSM-5 substance use disorder diagnostic terminology because of its uncertain definition and its potentially negative connotation" (p. 485). Editors also introduced *behavioral addiction* to the text of the DSM-5 (p. 481) and although the term is intentionally left undefined, behavioral addictions are then characterized by compulsive behavior(s), functional impairment, withdrawal, and tolerance (APA, 2013).

Today, an increasing number of behaviors are classified as addictions, such as eating disorders, gambling, and gaming addictions (Thege et al., 2016), while other behaviors labeled addictions are done so more controversially, such as television binge watching or excessive texting (DeSola Gutierrez et al., 2016). Even further, many behaviors are often referred to as "addictions" with speculation, such as tanning, texting, or shoplifting (Thege et al., 2016). However, studies clearly suggest that a wide range of substance and behavioral addictions serve similar functions (Sussman et al., 2011), and there is growing consensus on the similarity of substance and behavioral addictions (Liese et al., 2020). Notably, the inclusion of these disorders has been the result of increasing evidence that these behaviors share clinical, neurological, and etiological, similarities to addictions to substances (Petry et al., 2018). Therefore, among researchers and clinicians, addiction is most commonly understood simply as a disorder in which an individual is markedly reoccupied with a behavior that initially provides a desired effect (APA, 2021).

The Landscape of Addiction Treatment Options

Several frameworks for understanding and treating addiction have dominated research over the past century and informed the landscape of treatment as it exists today. Most popular is the disease model, introduced in the late 19th century and supported by numerous studies, which posits that addiction is a physical disease based in genetic dispositions and abnormalities in the structure of the brain (APA, 2017; National Institute on Alcohol Abuse and Alcoholism [NIAAA], 2017). While the disease model should not be discredited, its treatment of addiction as a chronic condition suggests we should treat behavioral symptoms of a disease with no cure (Cihan et al., 2014). Treatment options available today are therefore largely evidence-based methods such as Cognitive Behavioral Therapy and Motivational Interviewing. While these interventions reduce symptomology and appear cost-effective, staggering rates of relapse and cross-addictions eventually prove these treatments to be costly in the long run (Fletcher et al., 2015; NIDA, 2019).

Meanwhile, psychodynamic treatments have historically been considered outside the scope of treatment for substance use (Trub & Campbell, 2018) and research regarding the use of psychodynamic approaches to address addictive substances or behaviors is sparse. Popular treatment models also do little to encourage relationship work in early recovery and couples therapy is often considered a form of treatment to be delayed until the partner in addiction has had time to prioritize individual treatment. Although a myth persists that couples work is counterproductive, there is no evidence to support this position. In fact, recent research has validated the fact addiction is, more likely than not, an issue of marriage and family (Godleski & Leonard, 2019) and involving partners or families of those struggling with addiction has been shown to produce a positive impact on relapse prevention and patient engagement (Slesnick & Zhang, 2016) and improve chances of abstinence (Chanel & Wesley, 2015).

Childhood Attachment and Addiction

In recent years, a growing body of research has begun to examine the relationship between attachment styles and addiction. Studies on parent-child attachment have established that a secure parent-child attachment is a factor of protection against issues of addiction (Cornellà-Font et al., 2018). On the other hand, childhood trauma and insecure attachment are known risk factors for developing issues of addiction including alcohol abuse, gambling, and substance abuse (Anderson et al., 2019; Delvecchio et al., 2016; Fridman, 2019; Keough et al., 2018) as well as eating disorders (Hertz et al., 2012), problematic Internet and social media use (Liu et al., 2016; Worsley et al., 2018), online sexual activity and sex addictions (Benfield, 2018; Bolshinsky & Gelkopf, 2019; Whoeler et al., 2018), and smartphone addictions (Kim & Koh, 2018; Xie et al., 2019). Addiction is also now known to be intergenerationally transmittable not only due to genetic factors, but because parental addictions negatively affect parenting roles and responsibilities such as bonding, supervision, and success, all of which increase the risk of substance use among the children (Fisher et al., 2016). This research again suggests that the development of secure or insecure attachment styles might significantly affect susceptibility to addiction. The well-documented and reciprocal relationship of addiction and relationship health is worth understanding with greater clarity not only to better understand the etiology of addiction, but the necessary evolution of options for the successful treatment thereof.

Adult Attachment and Addiction

Studies on adult attachment have similarly established that securely attached adults are better able to emotionally self-regulate with positive behaviors and use interpersonal contact in a close relationship to alter or stabilize one's neurophysiology in the face of stress (Mikulincer, 1998; Mikulincer & Shaver; 2012; Katehakis, 2017). On the other hand, insecurely attached partners are more likely to use dysfunctional methods to soothe, such as sexual addictions, alcohol abuse, marijuana abuse, and texting (Liese et al., 2020; Love et al., 2016; Molnar et al., 2010).

Meanwhile, intimate relationships such as marriage play an important role in the mental and physical well-being of individuals (Whisman & Baucom, 2012). In Western cultures approximately 90 percent of individuals will marry by the age of 50 and marriage has been shown to have a positive effect on the mental health of partner as well as their children (American Psychological Association, 2021). Being in a healthy, committed relationship reduces the risk of disease and increases lifespan (Holt-Lunstad et al., 2017). Relationship distress, however, has been shown to prime individuals for a variety of mental health issues including mood and anxiety disorders and, notably, issues of addiction (Bhatia & Davila, 2017).

Studies suggest addiction has destructive effects on close relationships (Fletcher & Macintosh, 2016; Gottman & Silver, 2012), a view seemingly integrated into the DSM-5 in listing interpersonal problems as one diagnostic criterion for problematic drug or alcohol use (APA, 2013). Addictive behaviors have also been shown to cause a decrease in relationship satisfaction (Whisman & Baucom, 2012). Although a significant association between insecure attachment and addiction is well established, the causal direction is still not well understood. A recent meta-analysis of 34 longitudinal studies (Fairbairn et al., 2018) found that while it has long been assumed that addiction causes relationship distress and attachment insecurities, in fact, the opposite might be true. Fairbairn et al. (2018) discovered not only that insecure attachment often precedes substance use, but that the path from early attachment insecurities to later substance use is significantly stronger than the path from early substance use to later attachment insecurities. What is more, insecure attachment preceded increases in substance use problems, regardless of the type of substance (e.g., alcohol, nicotine, or marijuana). Attachment insecurities have also been found to predict behavioral dependencies (Estevez et al., 2019). These studies suggest that however well-established this link between insecure attachment and addiction has become, further research is required to understand the causal direction of factors involved and consider the most effective approaches to treatment thereof.

Attachment Repair to Treat Addiction

If recent research suggests it is the insecurity of close relationships that precedes addiction (Fairbairn et al., 2018), and addiction might be treated through creating more secure attachment bonds to intimate partners, the obvious place to start would be in couples therapy. Romantic partners often become primary attachment figures in adulthood (Castellano et al., 2018) and for many individuals, a marriage or partnership will be the most intimate relationship during one's lifetime (Whisman & Baucom, 2012). From an attachment perspective, it is not until one is able to regulate affect and self-soothe with relationships that one will not require outside substances or distractions to do this task for them. High rates of relapse and cross-addictions (Thege et al., 2016) suggest that until secure attachments are achieved in life, relapse will occur or addictions will simply be replaced with another. Current research demands that therapists consider couples therapy as one valuable arena to address issues of attachment that may perpetuate symptoms of addiction. The expectation is that more securely attached partners will more easily remain balanced in the face of stressors so reliance on the addictive substance or behavior diminishes (Mikulincer & Shaver, 2012).

Despite the large body of attachment research in existence, however, no one model exists for an attachment-based approach to counseling. Bowlby himself avoided establishing a school of attachment-based therapy (Holmes, 2015), but he did set out basic principles to guide therapeutic tasks: (a) the provision of a secure base, which involves a therapist offering a patient a secure foundation from which they can explore past painful experiences; (b) the exploration of significant relationships, including past attachments and their effect on expectations and feelings in current relationships; (c) the exploration of the therapeutic relationship and how it relates to other relationships; (d) the linking of past attachment relationships or experiences to current ones; and (e) the revision of internal working models so that patients can begin to feel, think, and act in new ways (Bowlby, 1988). In therapy, a therapist might encounter several contradictory internal working models to address in order to foster new adaptive reactions. Levy (2013) also proposed a sixth principle, or that the therapist offers the patient a safe haven during times of stress. While this safe haven initially exists in the therapy room, it may eventually become an internalized source of safety the patient can access in the real world. The usefulness of these basic principles has been expanded into prototypes within the context of couples therapy (Johnson, 2009: Solomon, 2009) but we still have much to learn about how these therapeutic tasks are best utilized or their effect on treating symptoms of addiction.

Traditional Couples Therapy

Every couple will experience conflict and the majority of couples entering therapy will cite "communication issues" as their presenting problem. Therefore, in traditional couples therapy, the focus is understandably on communication skills and conflict reduction. However, research actually demonstrates that success in relationship will hinge not on the number of arguments couples have, the method of dealing with anger, nor the resolution of disagreements (Gottman, 1994, 1999). Rather, the critical factor that will distinguish successful from failed relationships is the ability to sustain emotional connection and reconnection following arguments. In traditional therapy, the focus on communication will leave attachment ruptures unaddressed alongside feelings of fear or mistrust that precede attack or withdrawal (Solomon, 2009).

Alternatively, according to the psychoanalytic therapist few couples actually have issues that hinge on communication. Rather, it is the difficulty each partner has in regulating feelings that leads to cyclical patterns in relationship as they try to resolve their own feelings with one another. The growing body of research linking attachment insecurity to addiction (Anderson et al., 2019; Benfield, 2018; Bolshinsky & Gelkopf, 2019; Delvecchio et al., 2016; Hertz et al., 2012; Fridman, 2019; Kim & Koh, 2018; Keough et al., 2018; Liu et al., 2016; Whoeler et al., 2018; Worsley et al., 2018; Xie et al., 2019) suggests that instead of focusing on communication skills or conflict reduction, couples should be encouraged to consider the useful goal of creating secure attachment. Rather than reducing conflict, human connection might be considered the antidote to destructive patterns in relationship, including addictive behaviors, and a corrective emotional experience rooted in attachment might be the vehicle to get there.

Attachment-Focused Couples Therapy

If the goal of traditional addiction treatment is abstinence, and the goal of traditional couples therapy is conflict reduction, then the goal of attachment-focused couples therapy might be to end cyclical relational patterns, including addictive behaviors, that serve as barriers to emotional intimacy. Humans are neurobiologically wired to need secure attachment bonds offering a sense of safety and emotional availability during stress throughout our lifetime. While attachment styles are shaped at critically early ages and remain remarkably consistent over time, research also demonstrates that attachment styles are malleable and can adjust, subtly or dramatically, depending on experiences and relationships (Mikulincer & Shaver, 2012). Attachment styles could be said to be set in sand, not stone, as studies demonstrate that insecure attachment experiences can be altered by positive experiences of empathy, unconditional love, and acceptance (Johnson, 2019). Neuroplasticity is remarkable and transmitter circuits in the brain can be altered by our thoughts, feelings, beliefs, and relationships (Doidge, 2007). Because the brain is adaptable and we form new synaptic connections throughout the lifespan, the reworking of defense mechanism and patterns developed in early insecure attachment relationships might become a critical goal of any therapy (Solomon, 2009). Although it is possible to alter the nature of attachment in couples' therapy (Greenman et al., 2019), more research is needed to develop clinical interventions informed by current research into how the brain and its cognitive memory affect how each partner will respond to the other's emotions and behaviors.

In more recent years, attachment theory has gained popularity as a blueprint for understanding romantic love (Johnson, 2008) and the emotionally triggering events that define relationship discord. According to attachment therapists, there are key moments in a relationship in which emotional disconnection will ignite negative cycles of interaction that leave partners feeling attacked or abandoned. These moments, when a partner feels betrayal or abandonment during times of heightened need, are understood as *attachment injuries* (Johnson et al., 2001; 2009). At the same time, there are critical moments of connection that also create new safety and bonding that serve to heal disconnection that might be understood as *attachment repair*. It is thus the experience of renewed connection and the restoration of trust that might lead to healing after injury (Solomon, 2009). Using an attachment focus in couples therapy, therefore, might lead a skilled clinician to interrupt these destructive patterns and replace them with emotional intimacy and increased attachment security, thereby reducing reliance on addictive substances or behaviors.

The recognition of cyclical patterns in relationship based on emotions is not unique to any one approach of couples therapy, but is well observed in a few arenas of couples work such as in Emotionally Focused Therapy (EFT) (Johnson, 2019b) and The Gottman Method (Gottman & Gottman, 2008; Gottman & Silver, 2012). While studies validate EFT as an effective approach for alleviating relationship distress based in neuroscience (Greenman et al., 2019), more research is necessary to understand its effectiveness in treating addiction (Johnson, 2019a). What is more, even with its fundamental focus on attachment security, EFT leaves many principles of attachment unaddressed, including the identification of anxiety and defense mechanisms or the management of very real somatic experiences of anxiety and core complex feelings.

ISTDP will differ fundamentally from EFT and other attachment approaches in its foundational focus on the restructuring of each partners' anxiety and defenses in real time. With consideration for how the combination of emotional experiences and anxiety due to attachment trauma leads to emotional dysregulation and the neurobiological effects thereof, ISTDP offers a comprehensive approach to managing somatic experiences that might block connection. While there is a scarcity of literature on ISTDP couples therapy, the richness of information explored within literature that does exist is a call to the psychological community for further exploration of this approach and its usefulness in treating symptoms of addiction.

ISTDP Couples Therapy

At its very foundation, ISTDP is an approach of attachment repair. Based on the notion that humans are wired for attachment, it is early attachment ruptures between a child and parent that will lead a child to experience intense and conflicting feelings that must be kept out of awareness by the experience of anxiety and employing defense mechanisms (Davanloo,1990). The goal of ISTDP, then, is to manage the anxiety while interrupting the defenses that keep a patient from experiencing emotional intimacy. As the therapist manages a patient's anxiety and interrupts their defenses in real time, the therapist encourages intimacy and thereby both enhances the patient's emotional capacities and strengthens the therapeutic alliance (Frederickson, 2013; Kuhn, 2014). While a study by Frederickson et al. (2019) demonstrates that incorporating ISTDP in inpatient addiction treatment will increase treatment retention and decreases relapse rates, more research is necessary to further understand the effects of ISTDP on addiction and comorbid issues.

Originally developed to treat individual patients in individual therapy, ISTDP is nonetheless effective in its application within group therapy or couples therapy (Have-de Labije, 2006) and has much to teach us about how attachment affects mental health symptoms. As in all psychoanalytic couples therapy based in attachment, ISTDP, too, will approach the dysfunctional and destructive patterns of a couple as rooted in each individual partner's unconscious intrapsychic core conflict dynamics (Have-de Labije, 2006). The more intense and frequent past attachment traumas that exist in each partner's history, the more intense unconscious complex feelings of transference, anxiety, and defenses that will present in the relationship. The goal of ISTDP in couples therapy, then, might be for a therapist to take each partner down a road to their unconscious complex transference feelings individually and with one another (Have-de Labije, 2006).

Today, there is a paucity of literature to shed light on the nuanced interactions of attachment healing that might occur when ISTDP is utilized in couples therapy. The few exceptions include several articles that are rich contributions demonstrating fertile ground for further exploration of how ISTDP can inform our use of applying attachment techniques in couples therapy. First, Marion Solomon (2001) described how ISTDP couples therapy might lead patients towards awareness of how childhood traumas lead to anxiety and defenses, both of which create chasms in emotional intimacy within relationship. It is the unconscious systems of each partner that both establishes and maintains emotional distance. It is thus a partner's willingness to explore their own underlying feelings, projections, and self-sabotaging behaviors might be necessary to work towards secure attachment.

Josette Have-de Labije (2006) then wrote about the use of ISTDP in couples therapy and similarly asserted that, as in all psychoanalytic couples therapy, the dysfunctional or destructive patterns of a couple coming in for help are best understood as resulting from each partner's individual "unconscious intrapsychic core conflict and its dynamics" (p. 34). It is the intensity and frequency of past attachment traumas in the patients' history that provide the conditions necessary for such intense unconscious complex feelings of transference, as well as the chronicity of anxiety, defense mechanisms, and nature and degree of patient's ego and superego. Have-de Labije outlined the goals of an ISTDP therapist in working with couples, as well as steps to achieve this aim through a series of 90-minute sessions with each partner individually or with the couple as a whole. These primary goals in ISTDP couples therapy include helping each partner to acknowledge their part, or their defenses, in their deadlocked interaction and then to relinquish them. As well as helping each partner unlock the unconscious and experience complex transference feelings and impulses which are related to their past traumatic experiences in order to work them through them. The therapist will also help each partner see how they transfer the perception of past important figures onto the partner, how their pattern of anxiety or defenses is used to suppress sadistic impulses, guilt, grief, love, and how this system is complimentary to that of the partner. According to Have-de Labije (2006) "repeatedly experiencing and investigating in each presence the unlocked impulses/painful feelings, related to past traumatic interactions, the link with the present interaction with the partner and working through will - idealiter - lead to resolution of the couples' problems" (p. 36). Notably, while in individual ISTDP therapy it is therapist who will function as the vehicle of transference, in ISTDP couples therapy the therapist will instead "take care that it is not the therapist but the other partner who will function as the vehicle for unlocking the transference system of his mate" (p. 35).

Most recently, Catherine Lockwood and Reiko Ikemoto-Joseph (2015) co-authored an article on collaborative efforts to bring the most effective elements of ISTDP into their work as couples therapists. They offered an overview of the approach and its most foundational concepts, suggesting which elements might be particularly useful in their integration into couples therapy. According to Lockwood and Ikemoto-Joseph (2015), two critical goals of ISTDP couples therapy that support attachment repair might be: (1) to work towards a systematic restructuring of a couple's patterns of anxiety and defenses, and (2) to do so while also positioning the therapist as a temporary transference figure who might "draw fire away from the partner under attack by redirecting it into the relationship with the therapist" (p. 29-30). This, in psychodynamic terms, is often generally termed "working in the transference."

The first goal of working towards a systematic restructuring of a couple's patterns might be achieved as patients experience in real time the patterns of anxiety and defenses that block vulnerability and emotional intimacy. Common defenses employed in couples therapy include criticizing, blaming, dismissing, explosive discharge, stonewalling, sarcasm, intellectualization, dismissal, playing the victim and, in the most extreme cases, dissociation. According to Lockwood and Ikemoto-Joseph (2015), one main advantage of ISTDP lies in its aptness to demonstrate in real time how the anxieties and defenses of one partner affect a couples interactions as illustrated here:

> For example, when Partner A begins to detail her frustrations with Partner B, the therapist can help both partners observe that Partner B's anxiety is being channeled into his striated muscles and sympathetic nervous system in the form of full body muscle tension and a dry mouth, which then results in the defenses of intellectualization and breaking eye contact, which he deploys in an attempt to regulate both his rising anxiety and his underlying feelings of anger and sadness . . . These precise, moment-to-moment interventions work

especially well because they keep the focus on what is happening emotionally in the room. The couple's anxiety and defense patterns can be directly observed by both partners with the help of the therapist and restructured on the spot. If skillfully applied, this approach has the advantage of doing real-time repairs to the couple's capacity to healthily co-regulate anxiety and complex feelings. Also, helping the couple to observe together their precise emotional and physical responses in vivo also allows them to see their problem from an entirely new, neurobiological perspective, which serves to interrupt their habitual pattern of attacking and then distancing from one another. (p. 29)

The second goal of ISTDP couples therapy might then be to position the therapist as a temporary transference figure who is willing to "take the transference heat" (Lockwood & Ikemoto-Joseph, 2015, p. 30). After all, couples will enter therapy with deep and intense feelings towards one another that might be rooted in feelings towards initial attachment figures. Exploring these feelings in a safe manner for each partner is difficult, so the ISTDP therapist might invite one partner to explore the physiological manifestations of core emotions while distinguishing between experiences of feelings, anxiety, and defenses (Lockwood & Ikemoto-Joseph, 2015). This mobilization of feeling towards the therapist might then be further explored and connected back to the presenting relationship symptoms. Meanwhile, the other partner should be reassured that they, too, will have an opportunity to explore their own their own distinct physiological and emotional experiences in turn.

Notably, Lockwood and Ikemoto-Joseph (2015) specified that it should be the therapist to "take the transference heat," a view that differs from that of Have-de Labije (2006), who urged that it should be the other partner who will be the vehicle for unlocking transference. The authors convincingly point out that while other psychodynamic approaches encourage an interpretation of a patient's feelings of transference, few approaches will so strongly encourage the therapist to step in the line of fire in order to explore a patient's barriers to emotional intimacy. Combined with anxiety management and defense restructuring, it is easy to see how this approach might break down negative relationship patterns and encourage affect regulation with one another.

Based on their research, training in ISTDP, and work as couples therapists, Lockwood and Ikemoto-Joseph (2015) not only succinctly highlighted the advantages of using ISTDP in couples therapy, but also underscore the paucity of literature on utilizing this complex approach with couples. Their article includes a calling for further collaboration in exploring the usefulness and best practices of this intricate yet effective approach to attachment repair. Because while each and every one of the aforementioned authors offer a rich and layered consideration of the usefulness of ISTDP principles in couples therapy, there is still much left to be explored in its effectiveness to facilitate attachment in couples therapy and the effects thereof on symptoms of addiction.

Summary

While a growing body of research has established a strong association between insecure attachment and addiction, the causal direction of this relationship is still not well understood. In fact, recent studies have demonstrated the path from early attachment insecurities to later substance use is significantly stronger than the path from early substance use to later attachment insecurities. If research suggests it is the insecurity of close relationships that precedes addiction, and addiction might be treated through creating more secure attachment bonds to intimate partners, then the obvious place to start would be in couples therapy. Although a body of literature has explored the possibilities of applying attachment interventions in the treatment of addiction issues, there is not yet widespread application of these techniques, no less in couples therapy. Based in attachment, ISTDP has been shown effective in individual therapy and holds much promise for use in couples therapy. An exploration of the experiences of ISTDP couples therapists might be one very critical

step in not only broadening an understanding of attachment repair in treating addiction, but the

ability to do so in the space where attachment repair might be possible, or couples therapy.

Chapter 3: Research Design and Methodology

The objective of the present study was to explore ISTDP as an attachment approach to treat addiction in couples therapy. This chapter will offer an overview of the methodology of this qualitative study, which utilized a phenomenological approach to derive meaning from the lived experiences of therapists working with couples in addiction using ISTDP, an attachment approach based in attachment. It will then outline procedures that were used in this study, including the sampling method, study participants, and data collection and analysis.

Research Design

This study used a qualitative approach aimed at producing knowledge about the experiences of ISTDP therapists who work with couples using an attachment approach, and the effects thereof on symptoms of addiction. The intent of this study was to expand the current understanding of treatment modalities beyond the individual behaviorally based treatment programs that dominant the landscape of addiction treatment today. By evaluating the experiences of study participants, the hope was to enrich the current understanding addiction as a disorder rooted in attachment and expand treatment options into the very arena that might improve secure attachment, or couples therapy.

The present study utilized a phenomenological approach to derive meaning from the lived experiences of ISTDP therapists who have treated symptoms of addiction using this attachment approach in couples therapy. According to Creswell and Creswell (2018), a phenomenological study is a design of inquiry based in philosophy and psychology in which a researcher will describe the lived experiences of individuals about a phenomenon and culminate in "the essence of the experiences for several individuals who have all experienced the phenomenon" (p. 13). In this particular study, in-depth interview questions were constructed to understand the similarities in each therapist's experience, as well as the context of issues that arise, and lessons to be learned from their experiences. The interviews were then transcribed, analyzed and coded before elaborating upon the essence of each theme (Marshall & Grossman, 2011). In an attempt to explore this phenomenon, the research questions this study sought to answer included the following questions: What are the perspectives of ISTDP therapists on utilizing an attachment approach to treat addiction in couples therapy? How do ISTDP therapists conceptualize the etiology and maintenance of addiction? How do ISTDP therapists conceptualize treatment goals for couples in addiction? How do the experiences of ISTDP couples therapists inform the use of an attachment approach to treat addiction in couples therapy?

Rationale for a Qualitative Design

The growing emergence of qualitative research has been historically met with resistance among more traditionally trained psychologists as mainstream psychologists tended to minimize the scientific value of qualitative methods in comparison to quantitative methods throughout the majority of the twentieth century (McMullen, 2002; Wertz, 2011). However, a growing interest in the qualitative approach within psychology alongside growing demand for methodological diversity has brought about renewed interest in qualitative design (Wertz, 2011; Haverkamp & Young, 2007). While qualitative researchers still remain a minority within the field of psychology, the publication of qualitative studies is ever increasing.

Qualitative research, within the discipline of psychology, refers to methodical and scientific practices aimed at producing knowledge about the nature of an experience. Quite simply, it is "the investigation of open-ended material and narratives by researchers or raters who describe dominant themes that emerge in the data" (APA, 2021). According to Levitt et al. (2017), "Qualitative research tends to centralize an iterative process in which data are analyzed and meanings generated in a fruitful, recursive manner, yielding results that gradually produce original knowledge of psychological life" (p. 3). Because the objective of the present study was to explore ISTDP as an attachment approach to treat addiction in couples therapy, a qualitative approach was determined the most appropriate method for generating meaning out of the study participants' lived experiences. The hope was that this inquiry would allow for an investigation into the nature of the experiences of ISTDP couples therapists. Themes that emerged from the data might then produce knowledge about how an attachment approach in the treatment of addiction may inform current practices in the conceptualization and treatment of addiction and the landscape of treatment options in existence today.

Population and Sample

The idea behind qualitative research is to purposefully select study participants that will most effectively assist a researcher in understanding the research question (Creswell & Creswell, 2018). Purposive sampling is one of the most common types of sampling when using a qualitative research approach and will be utilized in this study in order to explore an attachment approach in couples therapy to treat addiction.

Study participants were licensed therapists, counselors, and psychologists who utilize an ISTDP approach based on attachment to treat addiction in couples therapy. The sample for this study consisted of six licensed therapists who met the following study criteria:

1. A minimum 5 years' experience using ISTDP in couples therapy;

2. A minimum 5 years' experience using ISTDP to treat addiction;

3. A minimum 3 months' active engagement in working with at least one *couple in addiction*, as defined herein, over the past year.

Respondents were recruited for participation in this study by accessing professional networks of ISTDP therapists. An initial formal *Recruitment Email Communication* (Appendix A) was sent to this network and a *Recruitment Posting* (Appendix B) was posted on the Experiential Dynamic Therapies email list ("EDT-list") to provide information on the study as well as verify inclusion criterion for participation. As potential participants suggested more colleagues to contact, the network of therapists invited to participate grew. Once a therapist responded and verified meeting criteria for study participation, they were emailed the *Informed Consent* (Appendix C) that included consent for study participation. Interviews with each study participant were scheduled on Zoom at the study participant's convenience and the *Interview Schedule* (Appendix D) was emailed to each participant for review in advance of the interview.

Validity

Several existing threats to the validity of this qualitative study were controlled to the extent possible. First, as with any study using in-depth interviews, the data collected was subject to the intrinsic bias of human study participants (Creswell & Creswell, 2018). To manage this threat to validity, the researcher interviewed study participants in a similar manner, asking each to reflect upon their experiences using questions from the same *Interview Schedule* (Appendix D). While interviews occurred in the context of a formal interview setting differed from than that in the natural field setting, the researcher also ensured that each interview occurred with the same background setting on Zoom.

Second, threats to validity of the present study were inherent in the fact that data collected included online interviews, and study participants had varying access to, and familiarity with, online technology (Cater, 2011; Janghorban et al., 2014). Technological issues did arise when one study participant experienced connection issues and lag times that could have affected rapport and procured missed data. To control for this variable, the researcher made sure to troubleshoot the connectivity and waited to begin questions from the *Interview Schedule* (Appendix D) until a secure connection was established.

A final threat to the validity of this study was that there are certain distractions and challenges present in online interviewing that are not present in face-face-interviews, including the simple fact that participants are able to view themselves during an interview and may find their appearance distracting (Oates, 2015). Or there is a potential risk for lost data when compared to face-to-face interviews such as missed gestures or expressions that might not be as easily recognized over a screen (Cater, 2011). In order to control for this variable, the researcher noted gestures or expressions throughout the interview that might communicate information and incorporated these notes into the raw data for analysis.

Instrumentation

A phenomenological study such as this one will culminate in "the essence of the experiences for several individuals who have all experienced the phenomenon" (Creswell & Creswell, 2018, p. 13). In the present study, the researcher conducted in-depth interviews with study participants in order to understand the similarities in each therapist's experiences. Interviews involved unstructured and generally open-ended questions, all of which are listed in the *Interview Schedule* (Appendix D). An unstructured interview allowed the researcher to modify the sequence and wording of the questions while ensuring that the same content was asked of each and every study participant. This controlled for bias in the questions selected or the manner in which questions were asked. Interviews were then transcribed using online software and coded before elaborating upon the essence of each theme (Marshall & Grossman, 2011).

In qualitative research, the researcher is the primary instrument of data collection and analysis (Creswell & Creswell, 2018). Because there is inherent bias any researcher will bring to gathering and analyzing data, the researcher in this study identified assumptions, personal values, and experiences that might facilitate bias at the outset and conclusion of the data collection and analysis process. To further control for these biases, the researcher used quotes from various study participants to generate rich, thick descriptions to convey findings, including many different perspectives of study participants, even when conflicted.

Triangulation of data was one final way in which the researcher ensured the internal validity of this study (Creswell & Creswell, 2018). Data was collected not through one source alone, but through multiple sources, including interview responses, video recordings, interview notes, observations, and careful transcript evaluation. In this manner the researcher was able to establish support for themes based on several sources of data and differing perspectives of several study participants.

Data Collection

Data collection in this research study, a qualitative analysis design, involved in-depth interviews that occurred in an online interview format. The hope was to obtain a rich resource of raw data for analysis, including Zoom recordings and the transcriptions thereof, as well as interview notes taken throughout the process. All data was compiled and kept on a password protected laptop that was stored behind locked doors.

In-Depth Interviews

In qualitative studies, a researcher will often conduct in-depth interviews with study participants that involve unstructured and generally open-ended questions. These questions are limited in number but meant to elicit the opinions and perspectives of study participants (Creswell

& Creswell, 2018). While there are limitations and advantages to an in-depth interview, and consideration of both was imperative when selecting a data collection instrument, the advantages to the in-depth interview outweighed its limitations in the present study for several reasons. First, an in-depth interview was particularly useful because study participants, or ISTDP therapists working with couples in addiction, are not always able to be directly observed due to issues of privacy and confidentiality. Second, using an in-depth interview allowed the researcher to retain control over the line and direction of questioning, encouraging study participants to share historical information as well as their perspectives and opinions on the study phenomenon of attachment in treating issues of addiction (Creswell & Creswell, 2018). Finally, and most importantly, using an in-depth interview comprised of open-ended questions as a data collection instrument was ideal for purposes of this study because it allowed for study participants to become teachers and for the researcher to become a student.

In the present study, the in-depth interviews were based on a set of research questions developed after carefully considering existing literature on attachment and addiction. The interviews included an introduction, the main body of the interview, and a conclusion. Each interview took place on Zoom and lasted approximately 60 minutes. The open-ended nature of the questionnaire was meant not only for the researcher to gather information on the phenomenon being studied, but for the researcher to gather data from the study participants based on their expertise and encourage unscripted responses to optimize the depth of data collection and research findings (Mack et al., 2005).

Informed consent was obtained from all study participants regarding the nature of the research and their participation in the study. The *Informed Consent* (Appendix C) included authorization for Zoom recordings was signed and dated by each study participant, copies of which were retained by the researcher. Study participants were also made aware of the fact that participation was entirely voluntary, and they were allowed to withdraw from the study at any point in time. Finally, study participants were informed of measures taken to promote confidentiality and protect their own identity to the best of the researcher's ability.

Online Interviews

The most common method for data collection in qualitative studies is interviewing and recent advances in technology have made the online interview even more common (Creswell & Creswell, 2018). While there are limitations to an online interview, advantages to the online interview outweighed limitations to rend it an appropriate data collection method for purposes of this study. Online interviews allowed the researcher in this study to overcome obstacles to traditional face-to-face interviews, offering increased accessibility and flexibility to both researcher and study participants. Obstacles to face-to-face interviewing were removed, including time and financial constraints, as well as geographic location (Janghorban et al., 2014; Mirick & Wladkowski, 2019). Finally, rapport building, critical to successful interviewing, was more achievable on an online platform than in telephone interviews as the researcher and study participants had access to one another's verbal and facial cues.

Data Analysis

Data analysis within qualitative research is a process of information gathering that often occurs simultaneously with the data collection process (Creswell & Creswell, 2018). As interviews took place in this study, the observations and memos collected were also analyzed and ultimately included as part of the narrative in the final discussions and conclusions. Because the text and narrative data collected from individual interviews was dense, all of the information could not possibly be included in the final results of the study. Therefore, it was imperative to "winnow" the data (Guest et al., 2012) and focus in on various parts of the data while disregarding other parts in order to aggregate data into a smaller number of themes (Creswell & Creswell, 2018). The data analysis procedure in this study was a process of several sequential steps that allowed for taking a large amount of information and organizing and encoding the data for optimal analysis. This process of data analysis included the following steps as outlined herein.

Organization of Data

The initial step in data analysis was to transcribe each and every interview, type up all field notes created during the interview process, and sort the data according to the type and source of information. Online software for transcribing each interview available at Rev.com was utilized to expedite this rather tedious process. This initial step in data analysis allowed for the review and obtaining of a general sense of information gathered during the data collection process, as well as the meaning of such information (Creswell & Creswell, 2018).

Review of Data

The next step in data analysis was to continue reviewing data and reflect on its meaning. Creswell and Creswell (2018) suggest asking several questions that might lead a researcher towards identifying meaning in the data. These questions included inquires such as, What general ideas are being communicated by study participants? What is the tone in which these ideas are expressed? What is the overall depth and credibility of the information? As these and other questions were considered, notes were taken in the margins of each transcript to identify emerging themes and concepts to which the researcher could return in subsequent steps of data analysis.

Coding Data

The next step in data analysis was to begin coding data. Coding is the process of organizing data by categorizing segments of text gathered during data collection, segmenting portions of text into categories, and then labeling those categories with an *in vivo* term based on the actual language of the study participants (Creswell & Creswell, 2018). According to Tesch (1990), there are generally eight steps involved in the formation of codes that were followed in order to generate codes for this study. First, all transcripts were read carefully to get a sense of the whole of the data. Second, one interview was selected, and its underlying meaning was explored before the same was done for all interviews. Third, a list of all topics was created, and similar ones were clustered together. Fourth, this list was taken back to the data in order to abbreviate the topics as codes and notate the data with appropriate codes. Fifth, the most descriptive words for the emerging topics were noted and turned into categories. Sixth, each categorical code was abbreviated and the codes were alphabetized. Seventh, data material was assembled in one place and a preliminary analysis was performed. Finally, as necessary, the existing data was recoded.

Generate Descriptions and Themes

After coding the data, the next step in the data analysis was to generate descriptions of the study components and participants, as well as themes for evaluation (Creswell & Creswell, 2018). Descriptions included a detailed portion of text about the study participants and their experiences that were particularly useful in narrative research projects such as the qualitative study at hand. A small number of themes then emerged, each supported by several perspectives of study participants and evidence previously cited throughout the rest of the study. As themes emerged, additional layers of analysis were made possible as themes interconnected with one another to form a new narratives and offer support for theoretical models already in existence. Finally, themes were analyzed in the context of this study as well as other case studies in order to go beyond description and theme identification and form deep and complex thematic interrelatedness (Creswell & Creswell, 2018).

Represent Descriptions and Themes

The final step in the data analysis was to develop a narrative approach that conveyed the findings of the study (Creswell & Creswell, 2018). This included a discussion of several themes, including subthemes, and specific illustrations of each as supported by verbatim quotes and various perspectives of study participants. Following this discussion of themes will also be a discussion of interconnecting themes identified that emerged throughout the study.

Limitations

Several limitations present in the existing study will be addressed herein. First, as discussed above, there are limitations inherent in an in-depth interview. Information received was filtered through the lens of the study participants and therefore subject to inherent bias. In addition, there existed the likelihood that not all study participants were equally perceptive to the occurrence of the phenomenon being studied or that they were articulate enough to convey its presence (Creswell & Creswell, 2018).

Limitations to this study also existed based on the inherent differences in the subject participants. While all study participants were licensed therapists, they varied not only in the licensure they maintain, but in the level of education and training they received and the extent of their clinical experience. They also differed in terms of their skill and perception in identifying and articulating the constructs being examined in this study. To limit this threat, the researcher ensured that each study participant met certain criteria most relevant to the research questions being asked. These criteria for study participation included a minimum 5 years' experience using ISTDP in couples therapy, a minimum 5 years' experience using ISTDP to treat addiction, and a minimum three months' active engagement in working with at least one couple in addiction, as defined herein.

Ethical Assurances

All standard ethical guidelines issued by The American Psychological Association (2002) were closely adhered to in order to maintain the welfare, protection, and privacy of the human study participants. In addition, this proposal was evaluated and approved by the Institutional Review Board (IRB) of The Chicago School of Professional Psychology to ensure that the study adhered to ethical codes as required to maintain protection of its participants. All study participants were informed of the nature of the study, as well as potential risks and benefits inherent therein.

This study posed minimal potential risk to study participants or the patients they see in treatment. As noted below, extra precautions were taken to protect study participants and their patients from risks associated with breaches in privacy and confidentiality. Minimal risk of emotional discomfort existed for each study participant as they were asked to discuss personal experiences and feelings in working with couples with addiction. To minimize discomfort, each study participant was notified in advance to expect such questions and maintained the right to refrain from answering questions at any point during study or cease participation immediately. Either way, the *Professional Therapeutic Referral List* (Appendix E) was provided to each study participant and the researcher was readily available to discuss with study participants any aspects of the study or their experience.

Privacy and Confidentiality

Extra precautions were taken to protect the privacy and confidentiality of study participants throughout the study. Each study participant was identified at all points throughout the data collection process with a pseudonym and under no circumstances was the study participant identified by name throughout the duration of the study, or in any publication thereof, unless explicit written consent was provided. In addition, the data collected during the course of this study, which included Zoom recordings and transcriptions thereof, was coded and securely stored on the researcher's private computer which was password protected and kept in a locked location. If any dissertation committee member was to access the data, they were required to sign confidentiality agreements. If any files were to be passed back and forth between the principal investigator and dissertation committee, they were password protected and sent through the email system of The Chicago School of Professional Psychology. Finally, all data collected throughout the duration of the study, including Zoom recordings, transcriptions, and interview notes, will be maintained for a period of 5 years following the publication of this study, after which all files will be destroyed unless explicit written consent is obtained to preserve data for other uses.

Summary

The objective of the present study is to explore ISTDP as an attachment approach to treat addiction in couples therapy. This chapter offered an overview of the methodology of the study and a phenomenological approach that will be used to derive meaning from the lived experiences of therapists working with couples in addiction using ISTDP, an attachment approach based in attachment. It outlined the study procedures, including the sampling method, study participants, and data collection and analysis. The next chapter will then include an overview of findings that resulted from this phenomenological research study.

Chapter 4: Findings

The purpose of this phenomenological study was to explore the experiences of therapists and address the central research question, What are the perspectives of ISTDP therapists who utilize an attachment approach to treat addiction in couples therapy? The objective of this study based on in-depth interviews was to bridge the gap between research linking addiction to insecure attachment and the clinical application of an attachment approach to treat addiction in couples therapy. Six ISTDP couples therapists were asked questions from the same *Interview Schedule* (Appendix D). In exploring the similarities and differences of therapist's experiences utilizing attachment interventions, the goal was to offer a more nuanced understanding of attachment principles in conceptualizing the etiology of addiction and its treatment in couples therapy.

Study Participant Demographics

All study participants were licensed ISTDP therapists, two males and four females, who utilize this attachment-based approach to treat addiction in couples therapy. Each study participant had a minimum 5 years' experience using ISTDP in couples therapy, a minimum 5 years' experience using ISTDP to treat addiction, and a minimum 3 months' active engagement in working with at least one couple in addiction, as defined herein, over the past year. All six therapists were located within the United States and interviewed on a Zoom platform. The following summaries offer general information on each study participant in terms of licensure and training in ISTDP, but more specific identifying information has been withheld in order to protect the privacy and confidentiality of these study participants.

Therapist 1

Therapist 1 is a Licensed Clinical Social Worker who has worked as a therapist since 2015. He is trained in ISTPD and was supervised under one of Dr. Davanloo's original trainees since

2012. For the past 12 years, Therapist 1 has worked in community health and private practice until recently when he began working exclusively in private practice. He reportedly enjoys seeing couples because it's a change of pace from individual work and utilizes a different skillset.

Therapist 2

Therapist 2 has been a Licensed Marriage and Family Therapist since 2014. She has completed core training or certification in ISTDP, EFT, and Accelerated Experiential Dynamic Psychotherapy (AEDP). Today, she maintains a private practice and specializes in sexual addiction and couples work.

Therapist 3

Therapist 3 holds a PhD in clinical psychology and has been a licensed psychologist since 2017. He completed core training in ISTDP and maintains a full caseload in private practice while also supervising both masters and doctoral level interns in the application of ISTDP. In his practice he sees primarily individuals and some couples, and he reportedly enjoys working with couples because he likes the variety in practice.

Therapist 4

Therapist 4 has been a Licensed Clinical Social Worker since 2006. She has completed core training in ISTDP as well as one year of advanced supervision in ISTDP and is currently in advanced training. Although her original career goals included working with individuals, she began seeing couples in 2014 and has continued to do so ever since. She enjoys learning about attachment and relationships and reportedly maintains a "pro-relationship stance" even in her work with individual patients.

Therapist 5

Therapist 5 has been a Licensed Marriage and Family Therapist since 2014. Prior to working exclusively in private practice, Therapist 5 worked in intensive outpatient substance use treatment centers, addiction treatment center for adolescents, and residential treatment for comorbidity of substance abuse. She then enrolled in ISTDP core training and today maintains a caseload comprised of both individuals and couples.

Therapist 6

Therapist 6 is a Licensed Marriage and Family Therapist whose experience includes over 10 years of working with individuals and couples using ISTDP and other attachment-based approaches. Therapist 6 offers a client-centered approach to treatment. She tailors interventions specifically to the individuals and couples she sees in her caseload in private practice today.

Results

This section will present the key results from in-depth interviews with the six study participants described above. Responses to the interview questions reflected differences in training and clinical experience, but also similarities in conceptualizing the etiology and treatment of addiction with its biopsychosocial roots in attachment. During this iterative process, interviews were recorded and transcribed using an online software, with the consent of each study participant, in ordder to ensure the accuracy and integrity of the information obtained. The researcher reviewed each interview thoroughly before labeling the interview content with codes and identifying emerging themes throughout the data. Each study participant was identified by a pseudonym throughout the study to protect their privacy and confidentiality.

After coding the data, descriptions of the study components and themes for study were generated (Creswell & Creswell, 2018). A small number of themes emerged, each supported by many, if not all, perspectives of study participants and evidence cited throughout the study. As themes emerged, connections were forged between themes (Smith & Osborn, 2008) and additional layers of analysis were also made possible as themes interconnected with one another to form new narratives and offer support for theoretical models already in existence (Creswell & Creswell, 2018). Finally, raw data was organized and clustered into five superordinate themes and 15 subordinate themes as detailed in *Table 1*. Each superordinate and subordinate theme will be introduced and described in a detailed narrative supported with verbatim quotes and clinical illustrations taken from interviews with study participants. In this manner, study participants themselves maintain a presence in the data and findings produced (Smith & Osborn, 2008).

As transcript interviews were reviewed and coded, many themes emerged that were common to the responses of all six therapist study participants, while other themes were unique to one or two study participants. As suggested by Smith and Osborn (2008), themes were not selected based purely on their reoccurrence within the interview data, but also on the richness of the passages from which these themes emerged, and their ability to illuminate other nuanced concepts from within the data. Each theme included herein brought about new insight on the complicated connection between attachment and addiction. Also included within the description of each superordinate theme is a description of the essence of that theme, which was drawn from a combination of the raw data and the researcher's interpretation thereof, creating an overall understanding of the "essence" of the experience of study participants as a critical component of this qualitative phenomenological research (Creswell, 2013). The following *Table 1. Superordinate and Subordinate Themes* offers an overview of these themes with superordinate themes and subordinate themes organized together.

Table 1

Superordinate and Subordinate Themes

Superordinate and subordinate themes

1. **Addictive behaviors are a defense on the triangle of conflict against feeling**
   1.1 Addictive behaviors are a syntonic and valuable defense against feeling that cannot be tolerated
   1.2 Addictive behaviors are a defense adopted in the wake of attachment trauma
   1.3 Addictive behaviors present in couples with low ego adaptive capacity

2. **Addictive behaviors are rooted in insecure attachment**
   2.1 Addictive behaviors are attachment reenactments
   2.2 Addictive behaviors serve a neurobiological function similar to attachment

3. **Defenses become the presenting problem in relationship**
   1.1 The intrapsychic becomes the interpersonal
   1.2 Addictive behaviors are a costly defense perpetuating insecure attachment
   1.3 Addictive behaviors are maintained by both partners in relationship

4. **Defense restructuring lays the foundation for attachment healing**
   4.1 Monitoring anxiety with rise of feeling in each partner
   4.2 Individual defense restructuring as necessary for heavy defense mechanism such as addiction
   4.3 Privileging the will of each individual partner
   4.4 Building capacity for feeling

5. **Couples therapy is a unique space to treat symptoms of addiction**
   5.1 Couples therapy is a unique space for attachment healing
   5.2 Restructuring defenses to build affect tolerance in couples therapy lays the foundation for secure attachment
   5.3 Secure attachment lessens reliance on addictive behaviors as a defense

Theme 1: Addictive Behaviors are a Defense on the Triangle of Conflict

All six study participant therapists conceptualized addictive behaviors as a defense on the triangle of conflict. The three subordinate themes to emerge included:

1. Addictive behaviors are a syntonic and valuable defense against feeling that cannot be tolerated;

2. Addictive behaviors are a defense adopted in the wake of attachment trauma; and

3. Addictive behaviors present in couples with low ego adaptive capacity.

The "essence" of this theme was that addictive behaviors are a defense against feeling inextricably intertwined with early attachment trauma, often leading to the formation of relationships with low ego adaptive capacity. The triangle of conflict, or the ISTDP model of intrapsychic causality, suggests that core emotions that are unrecognized or conflicted cause anxiety, which a patient then discharges through the use of a defense mechanism. Without a parent or caregiver available or able to attune to their emotional needs, an individual will adopt a set of behaviors to stave off anxiety and manage internal affect. These children who continue to employ maladaptive defense mechanisms as they grow in order to manage low tolerance for feeling in intimate relationships then end up in relationships where addiction is present to manage that affect.

1.1 Addictive behaviors are a syntonic and valuable defense against feeling that cannot be tolerated

The first subordinate theme to emerge mentioned by all six study participants was that addictive behaviors are a syntonic, valuable, and powerfully motivated defense against feeling that cannot be tolerated. Defenses are highly syntonic, or seamlessly incorporated into a character structure, when the defense holds great value, such as an avoidance strategy allowing for distancing amidst complicated or conflicted feelings.

According to Therapist 1:

I conceptualize the etiology of addiction as primarily a defense mechanism . . . Meaning that you engage in the addictive behavior as a way of managing anxiety and staving off things you don't want to face on the inside, whether that be heartbreak or grief or homicidal rage or excruciating guilt. But whatever it is, you're avoiding facing something by engaging the addiction. So it's an avoidance strategy, ultimately.

It all comes down to what we call the triangle of conflict. So that, that's a model for intrapsychic causality. Meaning that, uh, certain feelings and impulses, uh, are anxiety provoking. So let's say you have the impulse to, uh, choke your boyfriend or girlfriend, or lash out aggressively or whatever that creates anxiety. And then we use defenses to manage that anxiety and push the feelings outside of conscious awareness, or it doesn't have to be anger. It could be tender feelings, or it could be sexual feelings and impulses. But whatever it is, if we are conflicted around any of these feelings and impulses, we will get anxious when they begin to mobilize. And then we employ a series of defense mechanisms to manage the anxiety and push away the feelings and, and helping the people in my office see their own triangle of conflict and see how they're dealing with their feelings, and then helping them deal with them differently, that that's, um, that's the theoretical construct that I'm most conscious of.

[The patient] got some insight into the idea that engaging the porn addiction was what he did to avoid feelings about her not being as available as he would like for her to be. Like, the people on the screen and the porn, they're always happy to see him, they're always available. And so it's a way of covering up feelings about his wife not being available.

According to Therapist 2:

I use more of the ISTDP lens and seeing addictive behaviors are more of a defense against feelings and a way to regulate anxiety when anxiety gets high and emotions stir up, anxiety gets high and they want to escape.

According to Therapist 3:

I see addiction as, um a defense on the triangle of conflict. And I see it as a powerfully motivated defense because of its reward . . . Management of anxiety, um, dopamine or other neurotransmitter manipulation . . . and its effectiveness in avoiding emotional conflicts and traumatic memories.

An addictive substance or behavior is syntonic if they're continuing to struggle with it, meaning that in some way it works for them. And so unlike other defenses, which are more easily bypassed, they're more acutely problematic. Without a reward, these defenses are harder to treat because they often come with significant reward or effectiveness . . . So I assume the defenses are harder to work with, and I also assume that the feelings and anxiety underlying the defense are more significant or dysregulated or traumatic.

According to Therapist 4:

I view [addiction] as a, um, as a very complicated self-sabotaging defense . . . Um, it's a really effective form of self-attack.

Um, self-sabotage and punishment. I mean, I guess maybe that's the other thing is that . . . Oh, it's the rotating defense, that's the term. The cyclical or rotating defense that I, I think that alcohol or drugs also, um, they fit so many aspects of a defense. Like they, they fill in so many holes. You can use it to punish yourself, you can use it to punish other people, you can use it to escape reality, you can use it to escape emotion. You can use it to try and fill a hole, you can use it to try and actually connect more with other people on one level while putting up a wall on the other. You know, I mean . . . it just fits so many bills.

According to Therapist 5:

[Addiction is] anything we use essentially to avoid our inner world, our inner thoughts are intimate emotions. Um, the, kind of the, you know, escaping reality sort of thought process. [T]he addiction is, is essentially kind of what you do to escape, um, looking inward, looking at your feelings and kind of an avoidant, um, defensive strategy in a way.

> We get big feelings in relationship that can cause us anxiety, and that brings about our
> protective mechanisms or strategies. Those strategies can really start to get ingrained, too,
> in, in a, in a couple dynamic. And then you start to really feel like this is a familiar
> argument. This is a familiar, familiar . . . fight that we have over and over again.
>
> Um, and the more, you know, be just being in a relationship can stir up feelings of, of, you
> know, longings for bonding and connection and, and attachment . . . We're all wanting
> close, you know, connection bonding, attachment, and have that feel good, but that also
> stirs up, you know, a lot of different other feelings and can oftentimes create worried
> thoughts and . . . What are they going to think of me and what are they, you know,
> expectations in the relationship and . . . I kind of see it as, uh, people have longings and
> desires, um, and hopes, and then there are expectations that follow that.

According to Therapist 6:

> Addiction dissipates anxiety, but it doesn't regulate it . . . And addiction can be to a
> substance, it could be to a person, it could be to, you know, all kinds of things . . . So the
> addiction is the byproduct of dysregulated anxiety about complicated feelings inside that
> they can't hold.

1.2 Addictive behaviors are a defense adopted in the wake of attachment trauma

The second subordinate theme discussed by all six study participants was the powerful motivation to adopt addictive behaviors in the wake of attachment trauma in earlier life. Discussed among study participants were experiences of death, abandonment, physical abuse, sexual abuse, or emotional neglect by a parent. Also discussed was that these attachment wounds underscore a common experience of relationships being unsafe and a subsequent lived reality that is far safer to attach to an addiction than to other people. When asked about the correlation between earlier experiences of attachment trauma and addictive behaviors, Therapist 3 succinctly stated, "I would say it is closer to one hundred percent."

According to Therapist 3:

Typically the level of intensity of defense is correlated with the level of intensity of anxiety. And the level of intensity of anxiety is often correlated with the level of intensity of emotional conflicts. The level of intensity of emotional conflicts is often correlated with the level of intensity of trauma. Plus, the other way you could put it is the level of destructiveness of a defense is only tolerable if it's providing an equal reward, so equal relief. So why would I use an addictive substance or behavior that is incredibly destructive if it wasn't providing a unique capacity for relief? And why would an addictive substance be the only thing that can provide a unique capacity for relief? Well, either it's because of some intensity of anxiety such that no, you know, exercise or bath or self-soothing, self-care ritual, is sufficient . . . Or the level of detachment and dissociation that substance use gives me is what I need to overcome the intensity of the trauma that's coming up inside of me or that's flooding me . . . So that's where if somebody using such a powerful defense that is also powerfully destructive, it typically means they're only doing that without replacing it with a more adaptive defense or healthy defense when there is a level of intensity of need.

According to Therapist 2:

Lots of trauma. Lots and lots of trauma. Sexual abuse, verbal abuse, physical abuse, violence, uh, abandonment, death. Trauma, right? Like when children go through trauma and they don't have an attachment figure that can help them with their feelings, validate their pain . . . if we don't have attachment figures that can validate our feelings and give us a sense of autonomy, we, children will, you know, ignore themselves to stay attached. And that creates significant problems of insecure attachment, avoidant, um, preoccupied, uh, which is anxious. Um, so, or then, or the disorganized with a lot of trauma.

According to Therapist 5:

Attachment history is really important. Because what, what at least I've seen in some of my couples I've worked with is that those who struggle with addiction, um, you know, substances or behavioral, um, oftentimes have had kind of higher, you know, attachment traumas, or more, more kind of intense attachment traumas in their upbringing.

And depending on how they've experienced life and relationships, those expectations can vary greatly. So I think in her case, the expectation was that relationships aren't safe. They're not stable. Um, they're scary if you get close. And so the more that he would distance by going to porn, the more that it would kind of solidify that expectation in her mind that it's not a safe, safe relationship.

1.3 Addictive behaviors present in couples with low ego adaptive capacity

The third subordinate theme to emerge was that couples in addiction have low ego adaptive capacity. Meaning, quite simply, that their tolerance for feeling is low. Feelings tend to make them anxious and they discharge the anxiety by employing an addictive behavior. Also discussed by study participants was the fact that low ego adaptive capacity will make co-regulation among partners difficult. So the addictive behavior is adopted initially as a regulator of feelings, but unable to self-soothe, it is then inherently difficult turn towards a partner for co-regulation or soothing.

According to Therapist 1:

They all tend to have a lower, what we call a lower ego adaptive capacity. Meaning that often, uh, attachment traumas occurred earlier in life for them. And therefore, uh, they developed a, a more primitive set of defenses. Less . . . the, the defenses are less mature. Uh, they have a lower tolerance for affect, lower distress tolerance, lower, uh, reduced ability to contain anxiety in the skeletal striated muscle tissue that the anxiety is often channeled into the GI tract, or smooth muscle tissue, or what we call cognitive perceptual disruption. So the common denominator, the trend tends to be, uh, a lower ego adaptive capacity. But that can be, that can be, uh, strengthened. It's a muscle that can be built up.

According to Therapist 3:

Poorer anxiety tolerance . . . increased levels of trauma and emotional conflict. And less affect tolerance. And thus the need to have some significant defense to help them manage the affect that's there . . . A great way to put it, that the lower the ego adaptive capacity, the more destructive the defenses may be, or *need* to be, or the more destructive a person will allow them to be, based on the reward that they serve to compensate for the low ego adaptive capacity. Versus somebody who they can tolerate their feelings fine, they can tolerate their anxiety fine. Well, then they might not need to rely on a defense that also has destructive consequences like addiction often does.

According to Therapist 4:

A really difficult time with co-regulation. Like they really, when it came to regulation, they were really in parallel play. They did not have the capacity, um, to see what's happening with their partner . . . That all of them, they just were not noticing they're not using what's happening in their partner's face as any kind of clue about whether they should stop or go. And they, um, uh, just really had a hard time, even with my coaching, you know, of being able to regulate their partner . . . You know, the addiction starts out as a regulator [of emotion] . . . I think that's a hallmark of a lot people with addiction.

According to Therapist 6:

So another kind of principle is that clients don't, when relationships are going badly, they're not turning to each other for soothing in times of distress. And in fact, they're activating each other in times of distress. We want help them develop the skills to be able to soothe themselves and sooth each other.

Theme 2: Addictive Behaviors are Rooted in Insecure Attachment

All six study participants conceptualized addictive behaviors as rooted in insecure attachment. The two subordinate themes to emerge included:

1. Addictive behaviors are attachment reenactments; and

2. Addictive behaviors serve a neurobiological function similar to attachment.

The "essence" of this theme was that addictive behaviors are attachment reenactments based on relationships with our primary caregiver. In the wake of attachment trauma, then, the neurobiological underpinnings of our attachment system may require addictive behaviors to satiate a neurobiological need for connection. Also discussed was the biological need to be a primary in our most intimate relationships, suggesting that addictive behaviors may disrupt that balance by putting a partner in a tertiary position.

2.1 Addictive behaviors are attachment reenactments

The first subordinate theme, or that attachment re-enactments take place within a couple in addiction, developed as several study participants underscored the tendency to carry our blueprint for relationships into intimate partnerships in order to recreate past attachment histories. Whatever one does to themselff by employing defenses, they invite their partners to do to them. Ultimately this exchange mirrors the same attachment relationship a patient had with a primary caregiver.

According to Therapist 2:

Like there's just lots of trauma that has never been resolved from the past, big feelings from the past that get activated and enacted in the current relationship. So people are repeating patterns and so forth back then, and they're playing it out in their current relationship today . . . Like if they're, if they're distant and looking away, they're enacting, you know, their history of attachment, shutting down walling off, looking away or getting anxious and scared, right? So attachment is very much ever-present in the room. And that's why we as therapists need to be safe, need to be reflective. Why I'm not going to be doing lots of challenges if someone is like getting sick in my room. So really holding the space to be, um, uh, you know, a safe, other attachment figure that they can both attached to where I'm not going to be critical, or they're not going to perceive me as being critical or blaming[.]

According to Therapist 4:

You know, attachment, the blueprint we got from our primary caregivers is the relationship that we're continuing with everybody out there in the world. Right? We're constantly . . . projecting our history onto everybody else. She saw that he was interacting with his, you know, disapproving mother when he was interacting with her. But she did not see herself as having anything that she could do about that, that it was all just his projection. It's like, well, no, you're actually really good at, at doing this. He doesn't have to work very hard to see his disapproving mother in front of him. You, you hand it to him.

According to Therapist 5:

They're coming in with a background of, you know, their own attachment histories, their own experiences, the, the way they relate to each other and, and themselves as well . . . So they come in with their own history and that just activates the other person . . .   The [attachment history] will really start to inform the way we attach to our partner and the way we, um, interact with our partner. So I'm always kind of taking a kind of an attachment history to understand, you know, each person's upbringing and how they have related to, to themselves and to other relationships.

According to Therapist 6:

Her partner is doing with her *exactly* what she's doing with herself. She's doing with herself *exactly* what the mom did with her. So it's, it's like the partners have enactments with each other . . . Part of the therapy is to help them see the enactments that get played out and to be able to observe that and not do a counter enactment, but to, to unpack that, you know, and see what's, what's . . . how they're behaving with each other.

2.2 Addictive behaviors serve a neurobiological function similar to attachment

The second subordinate theme that the attachment and addiction are rooted in the same neurobiological systems discussed by several study participants. One study participant spoke of addictive behaviors as perpetuating the underpinnings of insecure attachment, while another discussed neurotransmitter manipulation by both addiction and attachment. Another study participant elaborated upon the biological need to be a primary in our most intimate partnerships.

According to Therapist 1:

[Addictive behaviors] are seen as defenses. And those defenses actually, uh, lock in, you could say an insecure attachment style. The defenses themselves perpetuate, uh, all the, the, the underpinnings of an insecure attachment, basically.

According to Therapist 3:

I see addiction as, um a defense on the triangle of conflict. And I see it as a powerfully motivated defense because of its reward …. Management of anxiety, um, dopamine …. or other neurotransmitter manipulation .... uh, and its effectiveness in avoiding emotional

conflicts and traumatic memories.

Given that they are all patterns of defense, um, and that oftentimes the neurochemistry is

similar in terms of dopamine, whether it's behavioral or, you know, pornography or

gambling or a substance . . . the neuro circuitry and firing and reward pathways are all very

similar.

According to Therapist 6:

We have a biological need to be a primary, which means that we come first. We come first

before everybody else. So if the partner's putting the other person in secondary or tertiary

position, it doesn't work . . .   That's why, you know, often like polyamory, you know,

doesn't work . . . [i]t really is a case to our biology, that we are hardwired to want to be

number one for our partner and how we go about protecting that primary relationship.

But we have also these two drives . . . We have a drive to connect and belong, and then

we also have a drive for autonomy. And, and our differentiation is our ability to mediate

those drives within us in between the partners.

Theme 3: Defenses Become the Presenting Problem in Relationship

All six study participant therapists that addictive behaviors, or any other defense employed,

as inevitably presenting as problems in the relationship. The three subordinate themes to emerge

included:

1. The intrapsychic becomes the interpersonal;

2. Addictive behaviors are a costly defense perpetuating insecure attachment; and

3. Addictive behaviors are maintained by both partners in relationship.

The "essence" of this theme was that addictive behaviors, initially adopted to manage intrapsychic conflict within one partner, inevitably cause relationship distress, disconnection, or primary relationship complaints. All of which perpetuate insecure attachment relations. Study participants also offered insight into the complex interplay of two triangles of conflict presenting in couples work, as well as the notion that both partners are complicit in maintaining insecure attachments.

3.1 The intrapsychic becomes the interpersonal

The first subordinate theme that the intrapsychic becomes the interpersonal was discussed by all six study participants. Or the idea that each individual maintains their own triangle of conflict to manage their interpersonal experience, but that while one might do so without interruption in isolation, problems are illuminated when one shows up in relationship. Ultimately, whatever issues a patient maintains personally, or intrapsychically, will inevitably present as primary complaints when a patient tries to connect with others in intimate relationship.

According to Therapist 6:

That's another assumption I have too, is that the intrapsychic always becomes the interpersonal. Whatever we're doing with ourselves then becomes the, um, portal to what's going on in the relationship...So if the client is using defenses that make them ignore neglect, disregard, um, rationalize, they're going to set up the counterpoint in their relationship.

According to Therapist 2:

You've got feelings that make you anxious and then you use. Right? Or you go have sex or go act out. Um, and, and this is between you and you. So she's always privileging the, the psychodynamics within the person and then how that gets played out in the couple.

According to Therapist 3:

Um, the triangle of conflict for each partner and how the various triangles of conflict are affected by the other partners, triangle of conflict. So how their patterns of anxiety and defense related to their feelings then affect the patterns of anxiety and defense related to the others' feelings. And how those can have reciprocal and sometimes compounding, um, effects in the relationship that lead to primary complaints that couples have.

When it comes to that theoretical orientation, um, my assumption or what I look for is the way the couple, um, responds to their own emotions and the emotions of the other. And how those patterns of responses to their emotions and the emotions of the other is the driving force behind their difficulties . . . Um, the triangle of conflict for each partner and how the various triangles of conflict are affected by the other partners, triangle of conflict. So how their patterns of anxiety and defense related to their feelings then affect the patterns of anxiety and defense related to the others' feelings. And how those can have reciprocal and sometimes compounding, um, effects in the relationship that lead to primary complaints that couples have.

According to Therapist 5:

We get big feelings and relationships that can cause us anxiety, and that brings about our protective mechanisms or strategies. Those strategies can really start to get ingrained, too, in, in a, in a couple dynamic. And then you start to really feel like this is a familiar argument. This is a familiar, familiar . . . fight that we have over and over again.

3.2 Addictive behaviors are a costly defense perpetuating insecure attachment

The second subordinate theme to emerge throughout the interviews mentioned explicitly by Therapist 1 was that with couples in addiction, "essentially that the maladaptive defense mechanisms are perpetuating an insecure attachments style." In other words, the cost of the defense

is emotional disconnection and, with the defense of addiction firmly ingrained with a relationship,

distance or enmeshment are maintained in a manner that does not allow for attachment healing.

According to Therapist 1:

I note the degree to which they avoid emotional intimacy. And to whatever a degree that

they avoid, emotional intimacy to that degree, they're not securely attached.

[Addictive behaviors] are seen as defenses. And those defenses actually, uh, lock in, you

could say an insecure attachment style. The defenses themselves perpetuate, uh, all the,

the, the underpinnings of an insecure attachment, basically. And so, uh, by disrupting those

defenses, by helping the, the couple, see how those defenses undermine their wellbeing,

undermine their communication.

According to Therapist 2:

Well, definitely, couples have a lot of, why they're coming to therapy, they're stuck. They,

a lot of, uh, you know, emotional disconnection between them, emotional distancing, so a

lot of hurts that they're not able to get resolved.

I think help helping the patient who uses active addiction to, to recognize that it's a defense

. . . against their emotional experience. And it's a way that keeps them escaped and, and

isolated from themselves and from their partner. And really pressing on the cost, you know,

to that.

I think it's incredibly important for them to know themselves, their feelings make anxiety,

make defenses. They can understand that, they can understand their partner, those feelings

make anxiety, make defenses. And then how do they see that both of their defense

mechanisms and strategies are, are causing their difficulties and their symptoms. Right?

Like helping them to see shutting down and going away and acting out is not promoting faithfulness, loyalty, security, support. The acting out behaviors, uh, especially with addiction, smoking, drinking, sex, what gambling shop, whatever it is, right? Is not promoting trust, safety, security. It actually is undermining what they both long for . . . ISTDP does a lovely job of helping the couple members to see that. Cause I don't think that's what pointed out in as explicit way of how them turning away and acting out and using is actually undermining the very thing that they wish that they had with themselves and with their partner . . . Cutting down, getting critical, shutting down all of these ways promote disconnection, not connection, not closeness. Right? It puts a barrier and a wall up and of course the addiction, yeah, they can have more, um, attention on the addiction than they do with themselves. So that would just show a disorganized attachment system or anxious or avoidant. All three can be in that category of addiction.

According to Therapist 3:

The addiction was with this one couple, the addiction was one way in which they keep bitter distance . . . By relating to substances as opposed to relating to each other. So I have a bunch of feelings about our relationship. Rather than experience and express those relationship for the purpose of connection, I will then manage those feelings by relying on a substance instead. So all of the feelings I have about the relationship are fueling deeper engagement with substances and then coping with substances and all of that.

So the alcohol was serving as a resistance to emotional closeness in ISTDP terms. And that in order to help them as a couple, we needed to not only block the, the alcohol addiction, but help them with the feelings that came with emotional closeness and the different reactions they then had to those feelings. Um, so underlying the alcohol addiction were patterns of projecting of splitting, of, uh, acting out of stonewalling of, um, threatening, uh

. . . all of these other things that the alcohol was blunting, for good, for good reason.

According to Therapist 5:

I think, for her to see that he could own up to that and see that there was something that,

you know, came before the affair. Um, and that's how maybe there was distancing in the

relationship already . . . Not to blame anybody, not to say that this is, you know, a shaming

thing, but again, it's so important to see how was, how were they turning away from each

other? Versus towards each other, uh, you know . . . Which then left them very suscept . .

. left him very susceptible, left, left the relationship susceptible to, um, more acting out,

you know, on this.

3.3 Addictive behaviors are maintained by both partners in relationship

The third subordinate theme that insecure attachment, and thus the use of addictive

behaviors, are maintained by both partners in relationship was mentioned explicitly by only one

study participant. Therapist 4 spoke about how often in her experience the non-addicted partner

often helps to maintain an insecure attachment. She spoke about couples tendency to have an

"identified patient" but in her experience, both partners are similarly positioned.

According to Therapist 4:

[T]he non-using partner was, *unaware* that there was an addiction problem until it exploded

. . . They're, they're interacting with a projection. They're not interacting with a partner . .

. And that's one of the things in particular with, you know, 'we've been married for 30-

some years um, and I had no idea.' And I'm like, 'Where were you? Where were you?

What, what was going on, you know?'

Where there's one there's the other. So frequently one partner looks a lot better than the other partner; that doesn't mean they're better, or I mean that they are more functional. That just means they're better at *looking better*.

Theme 4: Defense Restructuring Lays the Foundation for Attachment Healing

All six study participants conceptualized addictive behaviors as a defense that can be restructured to lay the foundation for attachment healing. The four subordinate themes to emerge included:

1. Monitoring anxiety with rise of feeling in each partner;

2. Individual defense restructuring as necessary for heavy defense mechanisms such as addiction;

3. Privileging the will of each individual partner; and

4. Building capacity for feeling.

The "essence" of this theme was that ISTDP couples therapy interventions involve anxiety and defense restructuring in each individual as a critical first step to lay the foundation for attachment healing in the partnership as a whole. Interventions discussed included monitoring anxiety with rise of feeling, and defense restructuring of each individual all while privileging the will of each individual to turn against the defense and build capacity for feeling. Also incorporated in this theme was the notion that careful attention must be paid to the physiological nature of anxiety, affect, and interpersonal attachment.

4. 1 Monitoring the anxiety with rise of feelings in each partner

The first subordinate theme of monitoring the anxiety alongside rise of feeling, a hallmark of ISTDP couples therapy, was mentioned by all six study participants. Also highlighted was the uniqueness of ISTDP in monitoring the physiological manifestation of anxiety to reduce the very real effects of dysregulated anxiety in blocking emotional connection.

According to Therapist 2:

ISTDP is probably the more, more thorough and it has a theory of anxiety. Like striated, okay, muscle tension. If they're getting sick or having IBS going to gastro that's, anxiety's too high. If they're, if they're not able to think, and they're having cognitive perceptual disruption, you can't, you have to regulate, you can't just continue to press or move on. You know, like, and with couples, you have to look at both people and really, moment to moment, tracking and noticing their anxiety channels, whereas EFT and AEDP and the CSTAT, they don't even talk about the anxiety. They don't have a theory of anxiety… That's a missing piece.

According to Therapist 3:

Uh, but the pacing and the timing of interventions and how long to focus on different dynamics, um, shows up differently with couples. Because if you're working with one [partner] and then the other [partner's] anxiety spikes, and then they start to enact a defense, which is destructive to the relationship, you need to deal with that. So I might not be done working with the defenses of one partner, but I have to then shift and address the anxiety and defense in the other partner.

According to Therapist 5:

I think [monitoring anxiety within each partner] is a huge one because you have two different, you know, two different people, unique people in the room. And one can be, you know, uh, more in kind of the striated muscle anxiety. So, you know, contained in their skeletal muscular system where they get tense and tight, and another partner could be experiencing kind of the smooth muscle anxiety where they might be getting nauseous and they're not necessarily . . . Or, you know, the thinking might be going kind of fuzzy with cognitive perceptual disruption. And so when that's happening, you know, you have to kind of prioritize or privilege the, the person who has more of the severe anxiety happening to regulate that . . . So being able to monitor both of those differences there and regulate one person's anxiety to help them think more clearly and be more present was a game changer for me, at least.

According to Therapist 6:

So obviously when the anxiety is in striated, right, we've got that green light to explore feelings, right. And then when they're exploring their feelings while the anxiety is striated, they're kind of on the road to their goals. If the, if the anxiety goes into the smooth or CPD um, from the ISTDP perspective, the three common interventions that we use is, uh . . . recapping with them. You know, helping them walk through the triangle of conflict so they're seeing what we see.

4.2 Individual defense restructuring as necessary for heavy defense mechanisms such as addiction

The second subordinate theme of defense restructuring as a critical component of working with couples in addiction was mentioned by all six study participants. Interviews stressed the importance of individual work within couples therapy to restructure heavier defense mechanisms such as addiction before restructuring the couples' system as a whole. Defense restructuring included identifying the value or function of the defense, the cost of the defense, and then inviting the individual to turn against the defense.

According to Therapist 1:

One is, um, chipping away at the overall defensive structure by addressing the here and now, and helping them turn against their defenses in here and now, and really selling them on the therapeutic task of facing things rather than avoiding things. Like they have to cognitively buy into that paradigm. That life is going to be better if I learn how to face things rather than avoid things.

According to Therapist 2:

ISTDP is a wonderful model to kind of restructure the defense patterns and restructure the anxiety pathways so that they can actually feel and deal and relate to themselves, to their partner and to the therapist.

[The addiction] is of value because it helps them escape the pain, helps them escape reality. Helps them to, uh, regulate their anxiety that's high, helps them to yeah, escape the pain. And, and, you know, we, we, we can appreciate that. But then today, three kids later, you know, how's that working out for you with, with your spouse and three kids and a family and a job? Like we understand it worked back then to help you cope and escape, but today how's that working out for you, this addiction?

According to Therapist 3:

My conceptualization of the treatment of addiction is the same as the treatment of any defense: helping somebody see the defense, see the function and cost of the defense. …First is working with the defense and making sure it's syntonic – or dystonic – and making sure the patient is motivated to turn against it. Uh, then helping them see the function of the defense, in terms of managing anxiety about certain feelings. And then helping the person to tolerate or bear or experience without overwhelming anxiety, whatever those feelings are and then using those feelings in some adaptive form . . . and then to process the underlying feelings and memories so that they don't have to use the defense in order to not be acutely anxious.

Uh, but the pacing and the timing of interventions and how long to focus on different dynamics, um, shows up differently with couples. Because if you're working with one [partner] and then the other [partner's] anxiety spikes, and then they start to enact a defense, which is destructive to the relationship, you need to deal with that. So I might not be done working with the defenses of one partner, but I have to then shift and address the anxiety and defense in the other partner.

According to Therapist 5:

When there's the addiction present, there's so much shame there's secrecy, there's a lot of hiding in the relationship. And so being able to start to be so forthcoming and honest, although it's a scary thing, um, it's, it can start to, you know, weaken the walls of the defenses and . . . Start to kind of restructure the, the person and the relationship to say it's okay that I share this. Um, my partner, isn't going to withdraw, my partner's not going to go away or shame me.

According to Therapist 6:

My thinking about this is that the more each partner can face the feelings that they avoid and turn on their defenses and, and have their anxiety regulated, the more connected they are, the deeper their attachment goes. Um, yeah, that's, that's my kind of guide. So I've always thinking about, you know, how can I, as the therapist be the conduit to help the clients face the feelings that they've been avoiding all along, and then see how that allows the two of them to connect. They both have to do that work.

4.3 Privileging the will of each individual partner

The third subordinate theme of privileging the individual will of each partner surfaced as several study participants mentioned the need for an individual partner to turn against their own defenses in order to reduce symptoms before the couples' system can heal. In some sense, it was suggested that fostering a healthy attachment system among partners involves an element of differentiation so as to refrain from unhealthy attachment reenactments from the past.

According to Therapist 2:

It really, it needs to be in both people, a wish to get well, versus my partner wants me here, my husband, me here, my wife wants me here, my dog wants me here. Right? No. It has got to be both, people having a wish to get well, to not continue to do these patterns, and, and, and the ways of that brings distance and disconnection between them. Both people need to be on board, and when they are, and they're able to have corrective emotional experiences by turning towards one another and sharing express, you know, honestly how they're feeling or what they're noticing in their bodies. Um, you know, it promotes, uh, results. But it's got to be, you know, it can't be my will driving the therapy. It can't be one of them driving the therapy.

According to Therapist 3:

Some couples, couple therapies see things as all about a bond or attachment or connection and some privileged differentiation with attachment. So there's different ways in, in which people conceptualize attachment. But finding a balance of we're connected and we care about each other, but we're also different and your life is your life, and my life is my life. And so helping a couple navigate that. Where some couples might be entirely enmeshed and 'I can't tolerate you having a separate mind,' or 'I can't tolerate you doing what you're doing so you have to stop because I'm too anxious about what you're doing.' These are enmeshment or codependent or anxious ambivalent attachment dynamics. Versus maybe more too differentiated, which would be, uh, you know, we're detached, we avoid each other, we don't speak, we don't contact, all that stuff. Okay. They actually need less differentiation. But when it comes to addiction and the, and the, um, consequences of addiction, often things are too enmeshed because one person is trying to control the addiction in the other. And it's not allowing the addicted partner to actually see for themselves the consequences of their addiction.

So part of the process with couples work is to help them differentiate enough where the addicted partner can have their own issue with their addiction without merely being resistant to the other partners', you know, complaints, or whatever it is . . . Then that's where these things can start to look like parent-child relational dynamics which then can trigger their own responses. Now, now the addicted one who's in the child role starts enacting whatever the child dynamics were that they did with their parents. How that adds another layer of complication in the relationship, because there's all this parent stuff about will and defiance and autonomy and stuff that's now getting activated in the midst of the relationship as well.

And so part of the dynamic is, okay, how do we get two differentiated but connected individuals, who are on the same level, who are expressing their desires and wants, and needs and feelings with each other, but actually don't need the other to satisfy those needs or wants or feelings in order for them to be okay . . . So how can I let go of my need for my partner to be different so that I can actually allow my partner to wrestle with their own issue while still caring about the relationship and asserting myself, but without making my ability to be okay dependent upon the other person's overcoming of their addiction or

whatever . . . And that sometimes it's actually the process of this partner letting go of

control of the other person's addiction that is the first step necessary in that other partner,

um, actually building an internal will to, to change their addiction.

According to Therapist 6:

But we have also these two drives . . . We have a drive to connect and belong, and then we

also have a drive for autonomy. And, and our differentiation is our ability to mediate those

drives within us in between the partners.

4.4 Building capacity for feeling

The fourth subordinate theme of building capacity for feeling, and the anxiety associated

therewith, was discussed by all six study participants as a key component of healing attachment

systems and reducing symptoms of addiction. Involved in this therapeutic task was privileging

honest feeling within the couple and allowing each individual to learn to tolerate the discomfort of

raw and complicated feeling without getting anxious and enacting a defense.

According to Therapist 1:

The work that, that happens in real time is also designed to, um, what we call capacity

building. So it will strengthen their capacity to tolerate distress, to tolerate anxiety, uh, just

by encouraging them to reflect on their own psychology, their own process, their own

experience. You're substituting more regressive defenses for higher order defenses. And so

the, the real time work in the office does, uh, create a sort of a sturdier platform from, from

which they can tolerate, or the idea anyways, optimally, uh, they can begin to tolerate

abstaining from the addiction and then facing that distress.

According to Therapist 2:

Like if they slip up for whatever, we, we, you know, we want to privilege honesty and truth telling. And not denial and not hiding and not lying. So a part of the muscle that we're trying to build for addicts, especially in like sexual addiction and when it comes to couples is to promote truth, telling to promote honesty, that relapses are a part of it, but that they would be willing to share with their partner and that the partner can have their feelings and process that in individual, but also in the couples counseling.

According to Therapist 6:

Um, so both of them needed to develop ways of tolerating, anger, um, in keeping their anxiety . . . And build their capacity to be able to face those feelings inside themselves and with each other, um, instead of ignoring and going passive.

So part of the task is that we have to help the client build a bigger vessel inside themselves to be able to hold mixed feelings while staying in the striated muscle. That's, that's the big task in the therapy is can we help them build their capacity without going into smoother, CPD or into . . . um, so that they can tolerate more inside so that the, that the need for the substance or whatever it is that they're using becomes unnecessary.

According to Therapist 5:

I'm just thinking of, um, like creating a lot of transparency and honesty for this couple is, you know, key. And so even him being able to share, um, and own up to the porn addiction and that this has been a struggle. Um, that actually helped, uh, this female partner, yeah, this, this actually helped her, um, understand the, the affair more. And how . . . the affair, uh, was almost like secondary, you know, it was like a secondary response of the porn addiction. And so being able to kind of trace it back to, okay, well, there's other things kind of blocking and getting in the way of, um, being able to be honest. Like the porn addiction kind of came first and then followed the, the affair. So that was really helpful. I think, for her to see that he could own up to that and see that there was something that, you know, came before the affair. Um, and that's how maybe there was distancing in the relationship already . . . Not to blame anybody, not to say that this is, you know, a shaming thing, but again, it's so important to see how was, how were they turning away from each other? Versus towards each other, uh, you know . . . Which then left them very suscept . . . left him very susceptible, left, left the relationship susceptible to, um, more acting out, you know, on this.

Theme 5: Couples Therapy is a Unique Space to Treat Symptoms of Addiction

Several study participants conceptualized couples therapy as a unique and valuable space to promote the very attachment healing that might reduce symptoms of addiction. The four subordinate themes to emerge included:

1. Couples therapy is a unique space for attachment healing;

2. Restructuring defenses to build affect tolerance in couples therapy lays the foundation for secure attachment; and

3. Secure attachment lessens reliance on addictive behaviors as a defense.

The "essence" of this theme was that couples therapy is a unique space to heal attachment, and that attachment is a critical component of treating addiction. Specifically, the work of restructuring defenses in order to privilege honest feelings, first within an individual and then within the relationship, allows for a more secure attachment eventually allows for a lessened reliance on the addictive behaviors as a defense against feeling.

5.1 Couples therapy is a unique space for attachment healing

The first subordinate theme, or that couples therapy offers a unique space for attachment healing and treating symptoms of addiction, was mentioned by several study participants for two different reasons. First, because our partners' presence actually activates "big feelings" and gives rise to the very defense mechanisms we need to restructure. Second, because critical to healing from addiction is building a secure attachment with the one person with whom an addicted partner is going home.

According to Therapist 5:

We get big feelings in relationship that can cause us anxiety, and that brings about our protective mechanisms or strategies. Those strategies can really start to get ingrained, too, in, in a, in a couple dynamic. And then you start to really feel like this is a familiar argument. This is a familiar, familiar . . . fight that we have over and over again.

According to Therapist 6:

So another kind of principle is that clients don't, when relationships are going badly, they're not turning to each other for soothing in times of distress. And in fact, they're activating each other in times of distress.

According to Therapist 2:

Because they're going home with each other. They're like the treatment team versus me. I'm not going home with them. You're not going home with them. Right. So helping, like build capacity for relatedness and emotional closeness and eye contact, eye-to-eye, face-to-face.

I'm not going home with them, right? They're going home with themselves and they're going home with their partner. So the, the real work is, again, that autonomy and attachment. Autonomy within themselves of knowing how they operate and understand their feelings, make them anxious, how their anxiety pathway is, and the defenses that they use. And on this side of the street, and then being able to help restructure those defenses, restructure the anxiety pathways so that they can feel and deal while relating to one another.

5.2 Restructuring defenses to build affect tolerance in couples therapy lays the foundation for secure attachment

The second subordinate theme that restructuring defenses to build affect tolerance in couples therapy fosters a more secure attachment was mentioned by several study participants. Conflict resolution or symptom management were mentioned specifically to not be primary goals in working with couples in addiction, but rather that they might be a byproduct of a more secure attachment.

According to Therapist 1:

Um, conflict is unavoidable . . . So I don't aspire to ensure that they're never in conflict, but another assumption is that if handled skillfully, the conflict can be an opportunity for increased emotional intimacy.

He got some insight into the idea that engaging the porn addiction was what he did to avoid feelings about her not being as available as he would like for her to be. Like the, the people on the screen and the porn, they're always happy to see him, they're always available. And so it's a way of covering up feelings about his wife not being available. And so one, he got insight around that. But two, his needs for her to be available became more satiated as both of them dropped their walls and defenses. And so, as they were able to form a more secure attachment, there was less of a need to engage the porn because he was doing that to fill the void of what he wasn't getting from his wife. Not, not necessarily around sex actually.

But more, more of an emotional availability, like I'm happy to see you kind of a thing . . .

Specifically, it was based in an attachment approach because moment-to-moment, play-

by-play, frame-by-frame, in real time, I would point out to them what each of them was

doing to create an insecure attachment. Meaning what they were doing to avoid being

emotionally intimate with each other. …That all of these behaviors, whether they were hers

or his, were simply substitutes or replacements for openly and honestly expressing how

they really felt and then supporting each other's feelings. So she would learn to support his

feelings. She would learn to say things like, if that's how I'm coming across to you as

scolding you, no wonder you're angry with me. I can see what you would feel that way. I'll

have to work on this. Thank you for letting me know. And he would learn how to say things

to her. Like, I wasn't aware of being aroused by this other woman, but there's a possibility.

And either way, if that was your impression, no wonder you wanted to strangle me. Yeah.

Thank you for letting me know. I can see why you would feel that way. You're not crazy

for feeling that way. So the expression of their true emotions and then each of them

supporting each other's emotions, *even if they disagreed*. With whatever the contention

was, they could still support the feelings. And that's how I dealt with helping the couple,

turn a corner away from an insecure attachment into the arms of a secure attachment.

According to Therapist 3:

Um, without attachment, other interventions don't work…So partners without an active

attachment bond, won't use the interventions that can help them. That the motivation for

using the interventions or the motivation for benefiting from the interventions flow from,

from the attachment.

The goal of couple's treatment is more than just to stop, you know, negative behaviors or

to stop addiction, but that the goal is to foster a secure and thriving attachment bond, and

that the defenses are just one reaction to a disturbed attachment bond. And so to work with

the defenses, um, but to do so without losing sight of the attachment bond that is underlying

the defenses and to always help a couple, keep reaching for that.

According to Therapist 6:

My thinking about this is that the more each partner can face the feelings that they avoid

and turn on their defenses and, and have their anxiety regulated, the more connected they

are, the deeper their attachment goes. Um, yeah, that's, that's my kind of guide. So I've

always thinking about, you know, how can I, as the therapist be the conduit to help the

clients face the feelings that they've been avoiding all along, and then see how that allows

the two of them to connect. They both have to do that work.

5.3 Secure attachment lessens reliance on addictive behaviors as a defense

The third subordinate theme, mentioned by several study participants, was that fostering a

more secure attachment lessens reliance on addictive behaviors as a defense against feeling. When

asked about experience regarding the over are all effectiveness of using an attachment approach

in couples therapy and the effects on symptoms of addiction, Therapist 1 stated, "my observations

are that generally I tend to be quite effective." Therapist 4 discussed couples who were able to heal

a relationship ravaged with addiction and maintain long-term abstinence. Therapist 2 mentioned

many couples that have recovered from sexual addiction and betrayals in the wake of attachment

interventions.

According to Therapist 2:

I have a good percentage of people that have recovered, which is impressive. It speaks to their, you know, to their value of their relationship, their marriage, their children, grandchildren, etcetera . . . I've had wonderful success stories of people wanting their life back, not wanting to go to a prostitute, not wanting to hook up with whoever and get diseases and not wanting to be addicted to porn and, and how isolating that is.

According to Therapist 3:

Once you then address the underlying factors that are causing the defense, it has the possibility of being not only more effective, but then less relapse . . . Because the fuel for the defense has been resolved.

A more increased reduction in symptoms of addiction and a more enduring effect into terms of lower levels of relapse. And this is, this is consistent with other findings in ISTDP, which demonstrate higher effectiveness rates when compared to treatment as usual, lower dropout and relapse rates.

[ISTDP] is complex and very accurate to the complexity of attachment and relationship. And yet once we understand the basic roadmap of that, it allows us to be very, uh, precise in our interventions and very effective and then very, um, long-lasting in terms of the effect of our treatment. So it's complicated, but once we get it, then it allows us to be really, uh, much more effective.

According to Therapist 5:

Um, and then for the partner, um, to, to see how vulnerable that is and to be welcoming with that, and then let that, let the person in more. Um, once you start to get those kind of little micro-moments in there, um, there seems to be less of the desire or less of the impulse to, to turn towards addiction . . . Not that it can wipe it up, you know, wipe it out in one day, but that these small incremental, you know, close vulnerable moments help, uh, help the person not turn towards their addiction.

According to Therapist 6:

Those kinds of interventions help build the capacity in the partners. Um, and so the more that we can do that, the less they'll lead to depend on the substance, the less they'll need to depend on an affair. That they learn how to regulate themselves, co-regulate the partner, um, and then they're in just in a much better position to deal with challenges in life. ISTDP does really well, um, in couples is that the exploration of feelings I think go deeper and, and you can get a more impactful, emotional experience through the ISTDP.

So the idea is if we can help the client depend on our relationship or each other. Um, then they don't have to use the addiction as the defense, amongst other defenses. They can use the relationship for soothing.

Summary

The purpose of this chapter was to present findings from interviews with six study participants addressing the central research question, What are the perspectives of ISTDP therapists who utilize an attachment approach to treat addiction in couples therapy? In exploring the similarities and differences of therapist's experiences in applying ISTDP interventions based in attachment, five superordinate themes and 15 subordinate themes emerged as detailed above in *Table 1*. The raw data, including verbatim quotes from each study participant, illuminated nuanced concepts in the clinical application of ISTDP treatment and brought about new insight on the very complicated connection between addiction and attachment. As themes emerged, a combination of raw data and the researcher's interpretation thereof led to a description of the essence of each superordinate theme. The following chapter will discuss these findings in the context of existing literature and further explore the importance of attachment principles in conceptualizing the etiology and treatment of addiction in couples therapy.

Chapter 5: Summary, Conclusions, and Recommendations

The purpose of this phenomenological study was to explore the experiences of ISTDP

couples therapists in order to address the central research question, What are the perspectives of

ISTDP therapists who utilize an attachment approach to treat addiction in couples therapy? The

objective of this chapter will be to discuss findings previously presented and then place them in

the context of the existing literature as outlined in the chapters above. This chapter will also be an

opportunity to explore themes to emerge that were not anticipated based on the previous literature

review and to introduce new research not yet considered within this context.

Interpretation of Findings

Throughout this study, several themes emerged, each supported by perspectives of one or

many study participants. As themes developed, the researcher returned to the raw data to explore

codes and establish connections between themes (Smith & Osborn, 2008). Additional layers of

analysis were then made possible as themes interconnected with one another to form new

narratives and offer support for theoretical models already in existence (Creswell & Creswell,

2018). Five superordinate and 15 subordinate themes brought about new insight on the

complicated connection between addiction and attachment. This section will attempt to place these

themes within the broader context of existing literature, organizing findings in the same manner

as presented above with superordinate and subordinate themes discussed in turn.

Addictive Behaviors are a Defense on the Triangle of Conflict Against Feeling

The first superordinate theme to emerge, supported by all six study participants, was that

addictive behaviors are a defense on the triangle of conflict against feeling that cannot be tolerated.

Subordinate themes weaved together to create a narrative that addictive behaviors are a defense

against feeling inextricably intertwined with early attachment trauma and low ego adaptive capacity. All study participants considered substance and behavioral addictions as synonymous, an approach supported by research demonstrating both serve a similar function with clinical, neurological, and etiological similarity (Liese et al., 2020; Petry et al., 2018; Sussman et al., 2011).

Addictive Behaviors are a Syntonic and Valuable Defense Against Feelings That Cannot be Tolerated

Study participants viewed addictive behaviors as "a defense against feelings and a way to regulate anxiety when anxiety gets high and emotions stir up." Also mentioned repeatedly was the syntonicity of the defense, or that "[a]n addictive substance or behavior is syntonic if they're continuing to struggle with it, meaning that in some way it works for them. And so unlike other defenses, which are more easily bypassed, they're more acutely problematic."

This finding that addictive behaviors are a syntonic and valuable defense against feeling that cannot be tolerated is supported by the work of Edward Khantzian (1997). Khantzian was one of the first theorists to suggest that substance misuse should be conceptualized not as a pleasure-seeking behavior, but as one to seek comfort and contact when unable to tolerate one's own emotional experience. It is also aligned with literature on the ISTDP model of intrapsychic causality, or the triangle of conflict. This model suggests that core emotions that are unrecognized or conflicted will cause anxiety, which a patient then discharges through the use of a defense mechanism, such as addiction, as a regulator of internal affect (Abbass, 2015; Davanloo, 1989).

Addictive Behaviors Are a Defense Adopted in the Wake of Attachment Trauma

Study participants unanimously mentioned the need to adopt such a potentially destructive defense mechanism as addiction in the wake of "[l]ots of trauma. Lots and lots of trauma." When asked about the correlation between earlier experiences of attachment trauma and addictive behaviors, one study participant succinctly stated, "I would say it is closer to one hundred percent."

Study participants also mentioned a myriad of experiences that meet the threshold for attachment trauma, including experiences of death, abandonment, physical abuse, sexual abuse, or the simple unavailability of a parent in validating a child's emotional experiences. According to one study participant, "if we don't have attachment figures that can validate our feelings and give us a sense of autonomy, we, children will, you know, ignore themselves to stay attached."

This finding that addictive behaviors are a defense adopted in the wake of attachment trauma is aligned with Bowlby's (1977) original theory. Or that the child whose needs for physical or psychological safety are not met by a primary caregiver, will develop an adaptive set of strategies that, while successfully managing immediate distress, increase vulnerabilities to psychopathology and clinical disorders from depression to eating disorders and substance misuse (Delvecchio et al., 2016; Fridman, 2019; Hertz et al., 2012; Levy & Johnson, 2019; Madigan et al., 2016; Tasca & Balfour, 2014). It is also supported by the conceptual framework of ISTDP, or the principle that it is early ruptures in the attachment bond between child and caregiver lead to a myriad of complex and often undesirable feelings that are suppressed from awareness by anxiety and defense mechanisms (Abbass, 2015; Davanloo, 1989). Attachment wounds teach that relationships are unsafe and establish a lived reality that is far safer to attach to an addictive substance or behavior than to other people.

Addictive Behaviors Present in Couples With Low Ego Adaptive Capacity

Study participants discussed, either explicitly or implicitly, the existence of *low ego adaptive capacity* among couples in addiction. A term commonly used in ISTDP, this describes "a lower tolerance for affect, lower distress tolerance . . . And thus the need to have some significant defense to help them manage the affect that's there." Also mentioned was a "really difficult time with co-regulation" and "not turning to each other for soothing in times of distress." Unable to self-soothe, couples in addiction are also unable to reach out to a partner for the very co-regulation that might make reliance on the addictive behavior unnecessary.

This finding is aligned with foundational tenants of ISTDP suggesting that the earlier and more intense the experience of attachment trauma, the more paralyzed the ego will become in managing resistance and repression (Have-De Labije & Neborsky, 2012). It also supports a view of addiction within an attachment framework, or Flores' (2006) assertion that addiction is "a consequence and a failed solution to an impaired ability to form healthy emotionally regulating relationships" (p. 6). Without a parent or caregiver available or able to attune to their emotional needs, children will develop with low ego adaptive capacity and enter adult relationships with a tendency to adopt maladaptive behaviors to stave off anxiety and manage internal affect. These individuals and couples may later present for treatment as a couple in addiction.

Addictive Behaviors Are Rooted in Insecure Attachment

The second superordinate theme to emerge, supported by all six study participants, was the understanding that addictive behaviors are a defense rooted in insecure attachment. Subordinate themes weaved together to form the narrative that addictive behaviors are attachment reenactments. Rooted in the same systems, addictive behaviors also serve a neurobiological function similar to attachment and it is easy to see why individuals with insecure attachment relationships will find it easier to attachment to an addictive substance or behavior.

Addictive Behaviors Are Attachment Reenactments

Study participants discussed attachment as "the blueprint we got from our primary caregivers is the relationship that we're continuing with everybody out there in the world . . . projecting our history onto everybody else." Or "the defenses are just one reaction to a disturbed attachment bond." In discussing a clinical example, one study participant explained, "Her partner is doing with her *exactly* what she's doing with herself. She's doing with herself *exactly* what the mom did with her. So it's, it's like the partners have enactments with each other."

This finding that addictive behaviors are attachment reenactments is supported Bowlby's (1969) theory of internal working models, or that defense mechanisms once necessary for survival as children will be incorporated into a blueprint for future relationships. It also aligns with theorists suggesting addiction should be conceptualized as an attachment disorder outright. According to Flores (2004, 2006), it is the individual who finds difficulty in establishing safe intimate relationships who will seek alternative methods to self-soothe when distressed. Finally, it aligns with the ISTDP conceptualization of addictive behaviors as a defense mechanism necessary to tolerate intimate relationships when an attachment history has taught one that relationships are dangerous. Have-de Labije (2006) aptly describes the importance of ISTDP couples therapy as "repeatedly experiencing and investigating in each presence the unlocked impulses/painful feelings, related to past traumatic interactions, the link with the present interaction with the partner and working through will—ideally—lead to resolution of the couples' problems" (p. 36).

Addictive Behaviors Serve a Neurobiological Function Similar to Attachment

Study participants also discussed addictive behaviors as "a powerfully motivated defense because of its reward" in its "management of anxiety, um, dopamine . . . or other neurotransmitter manipulation." Highlighted was that "oftentimes the neurochemistry is similar in terms of dopamine, whether it's behavioral or, you know, pornography or gambling or a substance . . . the neuro circuitry and firing and reward pathways are all very similar." Finally, discussed was the "biological need to be a primary, which means that we come first." Or that "if the partner's putting the other person in secondary or tertiary position, it doesn't work . . . It really is a case to our biology, that we are hardwired to want to be number one for our partner."

This finding that addictive behaviors serve a neurobiological function similar to attachment is well supported by Bowlby's (1969, 1988) theory that humans are biologically wired for close and loving bonds with those who can ensure support, safety, and connection. As well as other studies demonstrating that secure attachment is linked with positive relationship functioning, higher dyadic satisfaction, and flexible functioning in relationship, while perceived threats to the attachment bond between partners creates psychological distress (Bowlby, 1969, 1982; Delvecchio et al., 2016; Kobak & Hazan, 1991). Finally, this finding aligns with studies highlighting the strikingly similar patterns of affective, cognitive, and behavioral responses to attachment figures as to addictive substances (Burkett & Young, 2012). In light of these studies, it makes sense that the psychological effects of close relationship bonds are similar to the neurotransmitter high emitted when one engages with the substance or behavioral addictions that have become so valuable in managing affect.

Defenses Become the Presenting Problem in Relationship

The third superordinate theme to emerge, as supported by all six study participants, was that defenses such as addictive behaviors become presenting problems in couples therapy. Subordinate themes weaved together to create the narrative that the intrapsychic becomes the interpersonal, as there are two triangles of conflict at play in any relationship as each partner experiences the feelings and anxiety that makes defenses necessary. It is in couples therapy, then, that the interplay of defenses emerge in the form of relationship distress or disconnection that perpetuate insecure attachment.

The Intrapsychic Becomes the Interpersonal

One study participant succinctly stated, "the intrapsychic always becomes the interpersonal. In other words, "whatever we're doing with ourselves then becomes the, um, portal to what's going on in the relationship." Another study participant explained, "You've got feelings that make you anxious and then you use. Right? Or you go have sex or go act out." She articulated the goal of "always privileging the, the psychodynamics within the person and then how that gets played out in the couple." Finally, another study participant stated the importance of conceptualizing how "the triangle of conflict for each partner and how the various triangles of conflict are affected by the other partners, triangle of conflict. So the manner in which an individual patient's patterns of anxiety and defense related to their feelings then affect the patterns of anxiety and defense related to the others' feelings."

This finding that the intrapsychic becomes the interpersonal is aligned with the theoretical framework of ISTDP, or that defense mechanisms, maladaptive to healthy emotional regulation, will begin to cause problems as the defenses constructed to protect against feelings lead to symptoms including undesirable behaviors and relationship distress (Abbass, 2015; Davanloo, 1989). It is also supported by the position taken by most psychoanalytic therapists, which is that few couples actually have issues that hinge on communication. Rather, it is the difficulty each partner has in regulating feelings that leads to cyclical patterns in relationship as they try to resolve their own feelings with one another (Solomon, 2001).

Addictive Behaviors Perpetuate Insecure Attachment

Study participants highlighted that with couples in addiction, "essentially that the maladaptive defense mechanisms are perpetuating an insecure attachments style." In other words, the addictive behavior will lock into place the insecure attachment behaviors that keep two partners emotionally disconnected and unable to experience attachment healing. Also noted was the fact that addictive behaviors are a *costly* defense, perpetuating relational conflict or disconnection as patterns become "ingrained . . . in a couple dynamic" and "you start to really feel like this is a familiar argument" or "fight that we have over and over again."

This finding that addictive behaviors perpetuate an insecure attachment is supported by studies establishing that while securely attached adults use interpersonal contact in close relationship to stabilize one's neurophysiology in the face of stress (Mikulincer, 1998; 2012; Katehakis, 2017), insecurely attached partners more likely use dysfunctional methods to soothe, including sex or excessive drinking (Love et al., 2016; Molnar et al., 2010). It is also supported by studies suggesting addiction has destructive effects on close relationships (Fletcher & Macintosh, 2016; Gottman & Silver, 2012), a view integrated into the DSM-5 which lists interpersonal problems as a diagnostic criterion for problematic drug or alcohol use (APA, 2013).

Addictive Behaviors Are Exhibited by Both Partners in Relationship

Study participants discussed the potentially critical assumption that addictive behaviors are maintained by *both* partners in relationship. One study participant noted that in her experience, "the non-using partner was *unaware* that there was an addiction problem until it exploded" and that the non-addicted partner is complicit in maintaining an insecure attachment, as "they're interacting with a projection. They're not interacting with a partner." In discussing clinical examples and the emotional absence of a non-addicted partner, she explained "Where there's one there's the other. So frequently one partner looks a lot better than the other partner; that doesn't mean they're better, or I mean that they are more functional. That just means they're better at *looking better*."

This finding that addictive behaviors are maintained by both partners in relationship is aligned with research demonstrating not only that the individual who is not taught to regulate affect through human connection will turn to addictive substances or behavioral processes to do so

(Benfield, 2018; Molnar et al., 2010), but that a cyclical relationship will develop as it is eventually the addiction, rather than a partner, that becomes a safe and secure base for the addicted partner. It is also aligned with Solomon (2001), who asserts that is the unconscious system of *each* partner that both establishes and maintains emotional distance. It is thus a partner's individual will to explore their underlying feelings, projections, and self-sabotaging behaviors that lays the foundation of working towards secure attachment.

Restructuring Defenses Lays the Foundation for Attachment Healing

The fourth superordinate theme to emerge, supported by all six study participants, was that defense restructuring in ISTDP couples therapy will lay the foundation for attachment healing. ISTDP interventions discussed included monitoring the anxiety with rise of feeling in each individual, restructuring defense restructuring of each individual, privileging the will of each individual to turn against the defense, and building capacity for feeling within each individual and then within the partnership as a whole.

Monitoring Anxiety With Rise of Feeling in Each Partner

Study participants discussed monitoring the anxiety alongside the rise of feeling in each partner as one critical intervention used in treating couples in addiction. In differentiating ISTDP from other attachment approaches, it was said that "ISTDP is probably the more, more thorough and it has a theory of anxiety." Also explained was, "EFT and AEDP and the CSTAT, they don't even talk about the anxiety . . . That's a missing piece." Study participants noted the importance of ensuring a partner has "striated muscle anxiety" as a "green light" to press on feeling, and also mentioned was the futility of proceeding with couples therapy if one or both partners are above an anxiety threshold. "If they're getting sick or having IBS going to gastro, anxiety's too high. If they're . . . not able to think, and they're having cognitive perceptual disruption . . . you have to regulate, you can't just continue to press or move on."

This finding, that it is critical to monitor anxiety with the rise of feeling in each partner, is aligned with research suggesting that a patient experiencing symptoms above threshold will have exceeded their window of tolerance and can no longer regulate anxiety in a healthy manner. It is this patient who might employ destructive defenses that prevent healthy emotional experiences in intimate relationship (Frederickson, 2013; Have-de Labije & Neborsky, 2012). This finding also highlights the fact that while most therapies aim to reduce anxiety, ISTDP will differ as the therapist becomes a biofeedback loop for the patient and encourages recognizing anxiety as a sign of feelings on the rise (Neborsky & Lewis, 2011).

Individual Defense Restructuring as Necessary for Heavy Defense Mechanism such as Addiction

Study participants discussed how "ISTDP is a wonderful model to kind of restructure the defense patterns and restructure the anxiety pathways so that they can actually feel and deal and relate to themselves, to their partner and to the therapist." This finding that defense restructuring within each individual is necessary for heavy defense mechanisms, such as addiction, is supported by the theoretical approach of ISTDP, requiring that early in treatment a clinician should address the defense mechanisms that keep a patient emotionally distant (Frederickson, 2013; Kuhn, 2014). It also supports the first goal of ISTDP couples therapy as outline by Lockwood and Ikemoto-Joseph (2015), or a systematic restructuring of a couple's patterns achieved as patients experience in real time the patterns of anxiety and defenses that block vulnerability and emotional intimacy.

Privileging the Will of Each Individual Partner

Study participants mentioned the importance of "building an internal will . . . to change their addiction," or that "it needs to be in both people, a wish to get well, versus my partner wants me here, my husband wants me here, my wife wants me here, my dog wants me here." While this concept was not addressed explicitly in the literature review, it is highlighted in literature on ISTDP as one critical component of the therapeutic inquiry. That is, an ISTDP therapist will establish that the patient's motivation to enter psychotherapy is within the individual patient alone (Coughlin, 1996/2018) and thereby privilege the autonomy and will of a patient to no longer succumb to patterns of maladaptive defenses.

Building Capacity for Feeling

Several study participants mentioned the necessary therapeutic task of "capacity building" in treating couples in addiction. Included in this task was privileging honest feelings and impulses within the individual, and then the couple, all while allowing each individual to learn to tolerate the discomfort of raw and complicated feeling without getting acutely anxious and enacting a defense. "Or abstaining from the addiction and then facing that distress." Another way it was articulated was that "the task is that we have to help the client build a bigger vessel inside themselves to be able to hold mixed feelings while staying in the striated muscle."

This finding that building capacity for feeling is a critical component to treating couples in addiction is aligned with the assertion by Lockwood and Ikemoto-Joseph (2015) that, "If skillfully applied, this approach has the advantage of doing real-time repairs to the couple's capacity to healthily co-regulate anxiety and complex feelings" (p. 29). Or literature suggesting there might be two vessels being expanded during ISTDP couples therapy in the treatment of addiction. First, there is the individual vessel of each partner who must build capacity to tolerate their own feelings without enacting a defense. Second, there is the vessel within the couple itself that needs to expand to tolerate distressing feelings within the relationship and one another.

Couples Therapy is a Unique Space to Treat Symptoms of Addiction

The fifth and final superordinate theme to emerge, supported by all six study participants, was that couples therapy based in attachment reduces reliance on addictive behaviors. Subordinate themes weaved together to create a narrative that couples therapy is a unique space in which to foster attachment healing. Restructuring defenses to build affect tolerance fosters a more secure attachment, and a more secure attachment lessens reliance on addictive behaviors.

Couples Therapy is a Unique Space for Attachment Healing

Several study participants discussed the fact that couples therapy offers a unique opportunity for attachment healing for several different reasons. First, because "I'm not going home with them, right? They're going home with themselves and they're going home with their partner." Second, because a partner's presence actually activates the other partner's attachment system and gives rise to the very defense mechanisms that need to be restructured, as "they come in with their own history and that just activates the other person." One study participant noted, "We get big feelings in relationship that can cause us anxiety, and that brings about our protective mechanisms or strategies. And in fact, they're activating each other in times of distress." Therefore, the cycles that are "ingrained in a couple dynamic" offer an opportunity to privilege feelings with "honesty and truth telling" so that they no longer cause the anxiety that needs to be discharged with defense mechanisms.

This finding that couples therapy is a unique space for attachment healing and treating symptoms of addiction is supported by Coughlin's (1996/2018) assertion that "Feelings do not exist in a vacuum but arise both toward and in reaction to others. There is always an interpersonal context to the arousal of emotion, even if only in fantasy" (p. 6). An attachment perspective also supports this finding and suggests that it is not until one is able to regulate affect and self-soothe within relationship that one will not require outside substances or distractions to do this task for them (Flores, 2004, 2006). Or finally, that high rates of relapse and cross-addictions suggest that until the secure attachment of an individual is altered, relapse will occur or addictions will simply be replaced with another (Thege et al., 2016).

Restructuring Defenses to Build Affect Tolerance in Couples Therapy Lays the Foundation for a More Secure Attachment

Study participants discussed how the therapeutic task of defense restructuring will lead to a more secure attachment bond. One study participant mentioned that "if handled skillfully, the conflict can be an opportunity for increased emotional intimacy." A clinical example discussed involved a patient with pornography addiction who "got some insight into the idea that engaging the porn addiction was what he did to avoid feelings about her not being as available as he would like for her to be" while "the people on the screen and the porn . . . they're always available." Ultimately, this patient's "needs for her to be available became more satiated as both of them dropped their walls and their defenses" and "as they were able to form a more secure attachment, there was less of a need to engage the porn because he was doing that to fill the void of what he wasn't getting from his wife."

This finding that restructuring defenses to build affect tolerance in couples therapy lays the foundation for a more secure attachment is supported by a body of research linking attachment insecurity to addiction (Anderson et al., 2019; Benfield, 2018; Bolshinsky & Gelkopf, 2019; Delvecchio et al., 2016; Hertz et al., 2012; Fridman, 2019; Kim & Koh, 2018; Keough et al., 2018; Liu et al., 2016; Whoeler et al., 2018; Worsley et al., 2018; Xie et al., 2019). It is also aligned with the neuroscientific perspective offered by Neborsky & Lewis (2011) regarding changes to occur in therapy as a therapist offers a biofeedback loop. Or that attentiveness stimulates synaptic growth as a patient learns to engage the cortex to separate anxiety from emotions, leading to a more 'attentive ego' so patients can pay attention to the somatic and cognitive experiences of anxiety and become curious about the emotions that underlie the anxiety. Ultimately, neural circuitry once damaged by traumatic experiences are restored as the patient has positive experience of exploring and tolerating feeling with a safe relationship.

A More Secure Attachment Lessens Reliance on Addictive Behaviors as a Defense

Study participants discussed attachment as one critical component of treating addiction, or that "without attachment other interventions don't work." Also discussed was that "the motivation for using the interventions . . . flow from, from the attachment." When asked about the importance of attachment interventions in working with couples, one study participant laughed aloud and inquired, "can you do couples therapy without [attachment interventions]"? Finally, it was said that "the goal of couple's treatment is more than just to stop, you know, negative behaviors or to stop addiction, but that the goal is to foster a secure and thriving attachment bond, and that the defenses are just one reaction to a disturbed attachment bond."

Study participants discussed how in their experience, fostering a more secure attachment within a couple lessens reliance on addictive behaviors as a defense. Regarding the overall effectiveness of using an attachment approach to treat symptoms of addiction, one study participant stated, "my observations are that generally I tend to be quite effective." Discussed were couples able to heal a relationship ravaged with addiction in order to maintain long-term abstinence, and recovery from sexual addiction in the wake of attachment interventions. One study participant said, "I have a good percentage of people that have recovered" and "I've had wonderful success stories of people wanting their life back, not wanting to go to a prostitute . . . not wanting to be addicted to porn and, and how isolating that is." Another study participant noted, "Once you then address the underlying factors that are causing the defense, it has the possibility of being not only more effective, but then less relapse ... Because the fuel for the defense has been resolved." When asked about long-term effects of a more secure attachment, one study participant mentioned, "reduction in symptoms of addiction" and "lower levels of relapse." He aptly noted:

> [ISTDP] is complex and very accurate to the complexity of attachment and relationship. And yet once we understand the basic roadmap of that, it allows us to be very, uh, precise in our interventions and very effective and then very, um, long-lasting in terms of the effect of our treatment. So it's complicated, but once we get it, then it allows us to be really, uh, much more effective.

This finding that a more secure attachment lessens reliance on addictive behaviors as a defense, is aligned with studies on adult attachment establishing that while insecurely attached partners are more likely to use dysfunctional addictive behaviors to soothe (Love et al., 2016; Molnar et al., 2010), securely attached adults are better able to emotionally self-regulate with positive behaviors and interpersonal contact (Mikulincer, 1998; 2012; Katehakis, 2017). More securely attached partners, however, more easily remain balanced in the face of stressors so reliance on the addictive substance or behavior diminishes (Mikulincer & Shaver, 2012).

Recommendations

Addiction is among the most pervasive of mental health issues (Thege et al., 2016; Sussman et al., 2011), highly associated with relationship distress and comorbid disorders (Bhatia & Davila, 2017; Whisman & Baucom, 2012). Most current treatment options available today are based on the medical model of addiction and focus on symptom management. However, high rates of relapse and cross-addictions (NIDA, 2019; Thege et al., 2016) suggest that traditional treatments are failing to address the biopsychosocial roots of addiction. While research links insecure attachment to addiction, there is a gap in the literature regarding the clinical application of attachment-based techniques in couples therapy and their effects on symptoms of addiction. The following recommendations for future studies are based on findings in this research and the potential to fill in these gaps as they exist in the literature today.

Further Research on the Neurophysiological Effects of Anxiety and Attachment

In recent years, attachment theory has gained popularity as a blueprint for understanding romantic love (Johnson, 2008). Today, both Emotionally Focused Therapy (Johnson, 2019b) and The Gottman Method (Gottman, 1993; Gottman & Gottman, 2008; Gottman & Silver, 2012) are popular approaches that focus not only on communication skills, but emotionally driven issues in attachment relationships. These approaches, however, leave many principles of attachment unaddressed, including the identification and management of anxiety amidst the very real neurophysiological experiences of attachment (Neborsky & Lewis, 2011).

This study demonstrates not only the futility, but the potential danger, of failing to heed the physiological arousal of anxiety amidst each partner's attachment system within couples therapy. ISTDP, unique in its theory of anxiety, has much to teach the greater psychoanalytic community about the importance of carefully monitoring a patient's somatic experiences in order to ensure a patient is not above threshold and to work within the optimal window of tolerance. Further research regarding anxiety in the wake of attachment trauma is necessary to support more comprehensive approaches to monitoring these experiences. Studies on the neurophysiological effects of anxiety amidst attachment might solidify education and tactical approaches helpful to clinicians in identifying and managing the experiences of anxiety and attachment trauma that block connection and perpetuate symptoms of addiction, as well as the somatic experiences of secure attachment that might make co-regulation possible.

Further Research on ISTDP Couples Therapy and Attachment Interventions in Couples Therapy to Treat Addiction

Despite the large body of attachment research in existence, no one model exists for an attachment-based approach to counseling. The usefulness of basic attachment principles have recently been expanded into therapeutic approaches within couples therapy (Johnson, 2009a: Solomon, 2009), but psychoanalytic communities still have much to learn about how attachment-based therapeutic tasks are best utilized, or their effect on symptoms of addiction.

This study was an attempt to fill in some of the gaps in the literature on the application attachment-based interventions that exist today. Further research is required to offer therapists a more readily accessible attachment framework for conceptualizing and treating the prevalent mental health crisis of addiction within the critical space of couples therapy. ISTDP is one approach that is based not only on attachment, but the neurophysiological components thereof. Originally developed to treat individual patients in individual therapy (Have-de Labije, 2006), ISTDP has much to offer in understanding how attachment principles can be used to inform the treatment of mental health symptoms. However, there is a lack of literature on the application of ISTDP in couples therapy. The few articles in existence demonstrate an exciting opportunity for further exploration of ISTDP couples therapy and its potential effects on a myriad of mental health issues, including symptoms of addiction. While this study further expands on such possible interventions, more research is necessary to inform the clinical application of attachment techniques in ISTDP couples therapy and understand their subsequent effects on symptoms of addiction.

Implications

This study examined the perspectives of ISTDP couples therapists who utilize an attachment approach to conceptualize the etiology and treatment of addiction. The objective of this study was to bridge the gap between current research demonstrating a link between insecure attachment and addiction and the clinical application of attachment-based approaches. Clinical implications of findings in this study provide a nuanced understanding of the biopsychosocial roots of addiction and offer new direction to therapists who assess and treat substance and behavioral addictions in couples therapy.

Addictive Behaviors Should Be Conceptualized as Defenses Against Feelings That Become Presenting Problems in Relationship

Several frameworks for understanding and treating addiction have dominated research over the past few decades, informing treatment option in existence today. Most popular among them is the disease model (APA, 2017; NIAAA, 2017), and while the disease model should not be discredited, its treatment of addiction as a chronic condition suggests we should treat behavioral symptoms of a disease with no cure (Cihan et al., 2014). Implications of this study suggest, however, that rather than treating addictive behaviors as symptoms of brain disease, substance and behavioral addictions should be treated as highly syntonic and valuable defense against feeling that cannot be tolerated. Substance use, sex, alcoholism, disordered eating, working, shopping, exercise, and social media, to name a few, are addictive behaviors that might all be conceptualized and addressed similarly as defenses necessary to tolerate intimate relationships when an attachment history has taught one that relationships are dangerous.

Implications of this study also suggest that it is these defense mechanisms, maladaptive to healthy emotional regulation, that will then cause problems as the defenses constructed to protect against feelings lead to symptoms including undesirable behaviors and relationship distress. The intrapsychic becomes the interpersonal, as it is the difficulty each partner has in regulating feelings that leads to cyclical patterns in relationship as they try to resolve their own feelings with one another. The individual unable to regulate affect through human connection will turn to addictive substances or behavioral processes to do so (Benfield, 2018; Molnar et al., 2010), and a cyclical relationship develops as it is eventually the addiction, rather than a partner, that becomes a safe and secure base for the addicted partner. The defense of addiction can thus be understood as having locked into place the insecure attachment that keep two patients emotionally disconnected and unable to experience the very secure attachment that might promote symptom healing.

The Focus of Addiction Treatment Should Shift from Symptom Cessation to Building Capacity for Feeling and Secure Attachment

Therapists treating addictive behaviors as symptoms of a brain disease naturally focus on symptom cessation, but the therapist whose primary goal is to strip a patient of a defense as highly syntonic and valuable as addiction will simply be opening the door to readily available cross-addictions. Implications of this study suggest that instead of focusing on symptom cessation, couples might be encouraged to consider the useful goals of capacity building and the creation of a secure attachment. Building affect tolerance, both within the individual and the couple, will lay the foundation for a more secure attachment. ISTDP couples therapy demonstrates that involved in this therapeutic task is effectuated by privileging honest emotion within the couple and allowing each individual to learn to tolerate the discomfort of raw and complicated feeling without getting anxious and enacting a defense.

A neuroscientific perspective offers insight into changes occurring in the therapeutic process as the focus shifts from symptom cessation to building capacity for feeling. Attentiveness stimulates synaptic growth as patients engage the cortex to separate anxiety from emotions, leading to a higher tolerance for one's own emotional experience. As both partners pay attention to their own somatic and cognitive experiences of anxiety and become curious about the emotions that underlie the anxiety, neural circuitry damaged by traumatic experiences might be restored such that both partners have positive experiences of exploring and tolerating feeling within safe relationship (Neborsky & Lewis, 2011).

Tolerance for anxiety and feeling within oneself will have profound effects not only on how one operates individually, but how one engages with a partner. Instead of getting anxious, flooded, and enacting a defense, a patient might be able to tolerate anxiety and feeling within. Once able to self-soothe, the patient who builds affect tolerance is eventually able to reach out to a partner for the very co-regulation that might make reliance on an addictive behavior unnecessary. Eventually, the rewiring of neurocircuitry might reinforce a tolerable and safe exploration of feeling and facilitate a newfound ability to offer and accept co-regulation from a partner.

Therapists Should Monitor the Neurophysiological Effects of Anxiety and Attachment

Humans are neurobiologically wired for connection. Decades of research have established that attachment relationships are how we regulate stress in the face of physical and psychological threat. Although traditional couples therapy focuses on conflict reduction and communication skills, implications of this study suggest that a critical component of couples therapy should be the regulation of anxiety pathways in the body as a patient engages in intimate relationship. The therapist who fails to monitor and regulate the neurophysiological symptoms of anxiety and feelings within the couples dynamic may be complicit in perpetuating cycles of disconnection that maintain insecure attachment and addictive behaviors.

Consider the therapist working with a couple in addiction. As connection or conflict within the relationship are addressed, feelings and anxiety will increase notably throughout the session when each patient's defenses are confronted or blocked. Imagine that one partner, able to experience a healthy level of anxiety in either the striated muscle or the parasympathetic nervous system, experiences deep sighing, tensing and clenching of fists, or fidgeting. Or they may present with a racing heart, sweating, or dry mouth. Either way, this patient is able to tolerate and explore the rise of feeling within their own body (Frederickson, 2013; Siegel, 1999), explore their somatic experience in real time, and safely be invited to articulate emotion while staying present to engage with both therapist and other partner.

Now imagine the other partner does *not* have such a similarly healthy experience of anxiety. For this partner, anxiety might manifest as in the parasympathetic nervous system, or the smooth muscle, presenting as gastrointestinal symptoms including nausea, dizziness, or diarrhea. Or this partner's anxiety may manifest in cognitive perceptual disruption as they experience incoherent or racing thoughts, tunnel vision, or other visual or auditory disturbances. The therapist who fails to recognize that this one partner has exceeded their window of tolerance will continue to pressure engagement. Unable to tolerate the anxiety this brings, this partner might get sick or simply go offline, completely dissociated or unable to focus. Without awareness they are over threshold, the other partner and the therapist may perceive this partner as avoidant or disengaged. Even aloof or disinterested in their partner's emotional experience. In reality, this patient may care deeply for their partner and relationship but are simply too anxiously activated by their partner's emotion to remain present in their own body and engage meaningfully with others in the room.

The couples therapists trained to monitor and regulate the neurophysiological experience of anxiety and attachment of each partner within treatment will do so before safely exploring a rise feeling within each patient. It is this skilled therapist who is able to accurately assess that both partners are operating within their own personal windows of tolerance. Only then might they proceed to safely exploring each partners' own intrapersonal experiences of feelings, anxiety, and defenses that might otherwise block connection and perpetuate addiction.

Couples Therapy Offers a Unique Opportunity to Restructure the Defenses That Perpetuate Insecure Attachment and Addiction

Popular treatment models do little to encourage relationship work in early recovery. Implications of this study, however, highlight several reasons to prioritize couples therapy as a unique opportunity to restructure the very defenses that perpetuate insecure attachment and addiction. First, the mere presence of a primary attachment figure, or a partner, will activate the attachment systems that give rise to the very defense mechanisms that need to be restructured. As one study participant noted, "We get big feelings in relationship that can cause us anxiety, and that brings about our protective mechanisms or strategies." Cycles ingrained in a couples dynamic will more readily surface in the presence of one another, offering both therapist and patients a unique opportunity to examine the very feelings causing the anxiety that often so desperately needs to be discharged with addictive behaviors. A therapist then might then work with the couple to observe their emotional and physical responses in real time, which "allows them to see their problem from an entirely new, neurobiological perspective, which serves to interrupt their habitual pattern of attacking and then distancing from one another" (Lockwood & Ikemoto-Joseph, 2015, p. 29).

Second, couples therapy is a critical space to treat addiction because it is the unconscious system of *both* partners that establish and maintains emotional distance and an insecure attachment. Couples in addiction often present for treatment having consciously or unconsciously labeled the addicted partner as identified patient, but a focus on the addicted partner and their symptoms alone will keep the couple stuck in the same patterns that perpetuate symptoms of addiction. It is imperative that *both* partners actively establish an internal will to turn against their own defenses that maintain both emotional distance and the ensuing addiction. It should be the responsibility of each individual partner to explore their underlying feelings, projections, and self-sabotaging behaviors. Then in addressing the defenses of each partner, a therapist might lay the foundation necessary to work towards building secure attachment and disrupting the addictive behaviors. Eventually, able to regulate affect and self-soothe within relationship, neither partner will require outside substances or distractions to do this task for them (Flores, 2004, 2006).

Finally, decades of research have confirmed that few factors have such profound effect on the individual human regulation of emotion as do close and intimate relationships (Bowlby, 1988). Because a romantic partner serves as a primary attachment figure in life, there is inherent value in establishing secure attachment within this relationship. While a therapist can indeed serve as a healthy attachment figure (Holmes, 2015), the therapist is not going home with an addicted partner. Through restructuring defenses to build affect tolerance in couples therapy, a couple might foster the type of secure attachment in the relationship most available and thus most critical to healing.

Addiction May Resolve in the Wake of Attachment Healing

Attachment wounds underscore an experience of relationships as unsafe and a lived reality that is far safer to attach to an addictive substance or behaviors than to other people. Implications of this study suggest that an attachment approach to treating addiction in couples therapy is an opportunity to alter that reality, offering long lasting improvement in symptoms. The work of restructuring defenses in order to privilege honest feelings, first within an individual and then within the relationship, allows for a more secure attachment that eventually allows for a lessened reliance on the addictive behaviors as a defense against feeling. As both partners pay attention to the somatic and cognitive experiences of anxiety and emotions that underlie the anxiety, neural circuitry damaged by trauma are restored as both the addicted and non-addicted have positive experiences of exploring and tolerating feeling within safe relationship.

If the goal of couples treatment is more than to stop addictive behaviors, but to foster a secure and thriving attachment bond, then the defense, as one reaction to a disturbed attachment bond, may resolve on its own. The goal is that as securely attached adults emotionally self-regulate with positive behaviors and interpersonal contact, reliance on the addiction diminishes. An attachment approach to treating addiction in couples therapy, such as ISTDP couples therapy, demonstrates how addressing factors underlying addiction in couples therapy offers the potential of not only being effective in reducing symptoms of addiction, but with less chance of relapse once the fuel for the defense has been resolved.

Conclusion

We live in an increasingly addicted society. With ever expanding accessibility to smartphones, social media, food, substances, and pornography, adults and children are living in a world in which attachment bonds to other humans are readily eclipsed, or even replaced, with bonds to substances and behavioral processes. Traditional treatment options are short term and behaviorally based, and a myth persists that couples work is counterproductive in early treatment. However, cross-addictions appear readily while relapse rates remain high, suggesting that the most popular treatment approaches are failing to address the root causes of addiction. ISTDP has emerged among psychoanalytic communities as one approach based on attachment, but literature on its application within couples therapy is sparse. This dissertation study considered the experiences of ISTDP couples therapists in clinical therapy who utilize an attachment framework for conceptualizing and treating symptoms of addiction. Findings in this study demonstrate that if the goal of couples therapy is more than to stop addictive behaviors, but to foster a secure and thriving attachment bond, then the defense, as one reaction to a disturbed attachment bond, may resolve on its own and with less relapse as the fuel for the addiction has been resolved.

ADDICTED TO LOVE

the goal of couples therapy is more than to stop addictive behaviors, but to foster a secure and thriving attachment bond, then the defense, as one reaction to a disturbed attachment bond, may resolve on its own and with less relapse as the fuel for the addiction has been resolved.